Early Childhood Professionals:
Leading today and tomorrow

Early Childhood Professionals: Leading today and tomorrow

Marjory Ebbeck TITC MA(Ed) MEd(Admin)
GradDipEd(TESOL) PhD
Professor of Early Childhood Education
de Lissa Institute of Early Childhood and Family Studies,
University of South Australia, Adelaide, South Australia

Manjula Waniganayake BEd(Hons) PhD
Senior Lecturer in Early Childhood Education
Department of Learning and Educational Development
Faculty of Education
University of Melbourne, Victoria

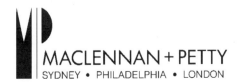
MACLENNAN + PETTY
SYDNEY • PHILADELPHIA • LONDON

First published 2003

MacLennan + Petty Pty Limited
Suite 405, 152 Bunnerong Road
Eastgardens NSW 2036
www.maclennanpetty.com.au

National Library of Australia Cataloguing-in-Publication data:
    Ebbeck, Marjory A.
    Early childhood professionals : leading today and tomorrow.

    Bibliography.
    Includes index.
    ISBN 0 86433 170 3.

    1. Early childhood educators.   2. Early childhood education.
    I. Waniganayake, Manjula.   II. Title.

372.21

Cover design by Manoja Ranawake
Index by Russell Brookes

Printed and bound in Australia

Contents

Leadership points from forward.

To lead
- An effective leader can help children become what they are capable of becoming.

- ECE have not accepted in the past they are leaders as historically they have been led by others.

- Learn to lead in order to help children fulfil

- ECE need to realise they are leaders + acknowledge they do this daily in the same way a CEO does. The issues they talk

- Need to understand Admin + Man in order to lead others. Not enough to know subject

- Leadership ideas meant to originated from other fields (as if ECE had no idea)

- Leadership is helping others to adapt to

Foreword

If I may be forgiven for paraphrasing the most famous English language author of all time, I would suggest that the central theme of this exciting book is: "To *become* or not to *become*; that is the question." Helping young children become what they are capable of becoming is what the field of early childhood is all about. And representatives of the field cannot fulfill their responsibility in this process unless they can function as skilled *administrators, managers* and, most important of all, <u>leaders.</u> This book offers valuable guidance to professionals who are willing to play all three roles and who desire to play them well.

Professionals in the field of Early Childhood Education and Care (to use the awkward term by which the field continues to be identified) have been loath to see themselves in these roles. Perhaps we have had something of a slave mentality: for so long someone else defined our goals, told us what to do and how to do it, and compensated us for our efforts by their own standards that it didn't seem to occur to us that we were capable of doing those things for ourselves. It is not an exaggeration to describe the field as having been inhibited by an overarching inferiority complex and to describe those of us who represented it as seeing ourselves not as we were but as a reflection of the way the general public saw us. Now that we have been "set free," we have not always known how to enjoy our freedom, how to set our own course, and how to achieve our own goals. This book reminds us that it is now our responsibility to do those things and offers valuable suggestions of how we need to proceed. If we are to help children become what they are capable of becoming, we have to become fully capable ourselves.

Although written by two distinguished early childhood educators, this book could perhaps be used as a text in a School of Business. With impressive erudition about administration and management issues, the authors introduce all the important concepts currently used to teach these subjects to business students and practitioners. Much of the literature reviewed comes from the field of management, and the reader has no difficulty applying these concepts to early childhood. It is rare that people in early childhood get there via the business route; rather, they get there because of their commitment to the development and welfare of children. However, once in the field, they find they need a lot of basic business skills to be able to do what they set out to do. They struggle with all the challenges faced by anyone starting or operating a small business. I think it is extremely helpful for early childhood professionals to realise that, when they talk about "high quality programs," they are striving to achieve the same thing as a CEO talking about "total quality management." Early childhood professionals, just as business leaders, need to understand administration and management in order to achieve quality.

It is in the authors' discussions of leadership that I consider this book most valuable. The two main professional antecedents of the early childhood field are education and social service. From the broad field of education came the "early childhood education" or "preschool" component of the field, and from social service came "day care or child care." Both of these broader fields fall under the umbrella of human service, even though education is more reluctant to accept that genealogy than is social service. It is interesting to note that early childhood per se has produced few if any of the "big names" in either of these parent fields; the course of influence has generally gone in the other direction. John Dewey, the great American educator, influenced kindergarten education, but it is questionable that any kindergarten educators influenced Dewey very much. Likewise, John Bowlby, the famous British psychiatrist who wrote compellingly about infant attachment, had a major influence on orphanages and child care (often assumed to be interchangeable), but there is little evidence that Bowlby modified any of his ideas on the basis of research or clinical information from the field of child care. Leadership in either ideas or practices was expected to come from outside early childhood, a clear manifestation of the professional inferiority complex referred to earlier. Furthermore, leadership that emerged from within the field was often strongly resisted. Ebbeck and Waniganayake make a strong case for the fact that this kind of situation can no longer be passively accepted. The field needs to produce its own leaders, and this book offers the outline of a strategic plan that will allow success in leadership development from within.

Effective leadership involves accepting the inevitability of change and helping staff and clients respond adaptively when it occurs. To quote the authors, "One thing is certain; the days of being insulated from change have gone, probably never to return." Heraclitus reminded us two centuries ago that we can never step in the same river twice. Certainly the field of early childhood is not the same river I stepped into over 30 years ago. Yet, paradoxically, people in this field—people who deal daily with the miraculous openness to change found in young children—can be strongly resistant to change. They often resist new ideas, new curricula, new procedures. Having personally experienced this resistance years ago when a few of us asserted that early childhood education was going to have to be re-defined to include (a) infants and toddlers and (b) child care, I still bear scars from the encounter. This book not only makes a strong case for the necessity of being receptive to change, but it also suggests helpful ways of involving staff and parents in the process. The book also reminds professionals in this field that they must become ever more socially and politically active. When sufficient numbers of effective leaders for the field have been developed, our collective influence will be infinitely greater.

The final kudos I wish to offer to the authors of this book relates to their emphasis on adopting a global orientation to early childhood and to encouraging leaders always to have eyes as this impacts on the futures of children. Most of us are shamefully parochial and regional in the professional literature we read and in the programmatic approaches we are willing to adopt. And yet the field of early childhood is truly a world-wide movement: what happens in Africa impacts what happens in Australia which in turn impacts what happens in Singapore, and on and on around the globe. All of these developments bear directly on the range of futures possible for children—for what they can *become*, as declared in my opening sentence. The movement has gained momentum globally for similar reasons: changes in cultural roles allowed women; new findings indicating the necessity of an appropriate expe-riential foundation during the early years for brain development, literacy, and academic progress; changes in patterns of family life; economic fluctuation and development; rapid development and dissemination of new technology; the spread of different religious orientations; war or peace between and among nations; protection or destruction of the physical environment; the maintenance of health and the transmission of disease. In short, to life. This means that we have to move out of the ruts of some of our concerns of the past—narrow debates about curriculum, age of enrolment, auspices for pro-grams, etc. What we are dealing with is the future of children, of ourselves, and of our planet. This book will help prepare a new generation of effective leaders in widely scattered geographic regions who can accept change, try to guide it wisely for the benefit of children and families, and in the process help early childhood earn the recognition it deserves as a field of significance and importance for human welfare.

Bettye M. Caldwell Ph.D.
Professor Emerita, Department of Pediatrics
University of Arkansas for Medical Sciences, and
Distinguished Professor Emerita, College of Education
University of Arkansas at Little Rock

Dr. Bettye Caldwell has been involved in the development of high quality early childhood programs in America for more than three decades. Her work in Syracuse, New York helped provide the foundation for Head Start. In Little Rock she launched and guided the Kramer Project, often described as a "school for the future." Kramer served children (and their parents) from six months through 12 years of age, providing full-day and year-round child care as well as education. Throughout her career, Dr. Caldwell's work has dealt with the role of the interpersonal and physical environment on the development of young children. Dr. Caldwell has conducted extensive research on the effects of early child care and has advocated for the development of a national system of educare (combining education and care) for children. She has served on many national and international boards and com-mittees concerned with early child development and has lectured on children's issues in more than a dozen foreign countries. She has received many awards in recognition of her work, including election to the presidency of the National Association for the Education of Young Children. In December, 2001 she received the Dolley Madison Award from Zero to

Three for "Lifelong Outstanding Contribution to the Development and Well-being of Very Young Children and Their Families." In addition to writing more than 200 professional articles and books, Dr. Caldwell has written extensively on family and child development issues for the general reader and has produced several educational films and videos. She recently moved into the internet age by becoming the early childhood specialist on the Fisher-Price Toy Company web site, for which she writes monthly articles and answers questions submitted by parents.

Acknowledgments

This book is the culmination of a collaborative venture that took place across two Australian cities, Adelaide and Melbourne. This presented interesting challenges along the way, especially when the technology broke down and the distances expanded to include international work commitments for both authors. Throughout the project, our families tolerated our being knee-deep in books and papers and permanently attached to a computer. Our heartfelt thanks go to our husbands and children for sustaining us with their love and understanding and allowing us the space and the time to complete this book.

Our sincere thanks go also to the professional colleagues who have supported this project in many different ways, especially in sharing their experiences and insight as reproduced in the text. Their interviews and case studies bring to life the diversity and richness of what is early childhood.

We wish to thank Lyn Conway for the diligence, tireless effort and expertise she brought to bear on the editing, formatting and presentation of the manuscript.

Special thanks are due to Fred Ebbeck for invaluable assistance in the reshaping of some of the content and for his editing guidance. Without his help the book would not have come to fruition.

Marjory Ebbeck

Manjula Waniganayake

January 2003

Leadership points from Forward

Introduction

This book is about leadership in early childhood. We believe that working in early childhood services is complex and challenging and that staff need both a theoretical and a practical knowledge base whatever their work role entails, be it as classroom practitioner, manager, advocate, policy maker or a combination of these and many other possible roles. The leadership role is particularly crucial if services are to survive and provide high-quality programs. In all parts of the world there are today increasing pressures to provide high-quality services, often with reduced resources, both physical and human. Standards of practice are being scrutinised and early childhood professionals are looking for support to manage in difficult times. Understanding theories and strategies assists early childhood professionals to address day-to-day challenges and at the same time be futures-oriented.

As early childhood professionals respond to the exciting challenges of the 21st century, we believe that they need to seek effective strategies to deal with change. They also need to understand the processes of policy making and how to influence policy decisions. This is what being a strong advocate for the profession is all about. Other contemporary leadership issues such as quality assurance, conflict management and mediation, partnerships with families and communities, advocacy for children and families, globalisation and futures are all on the early childhood agenda. To act proactively as leaders, early childhood professionals need to be well informed. This book provides broad frameworks to help professionals consider early childhood matters as leaders, viewing these from a global perspective into possible futures.

We have adopted an integrated approach to leadership in early childhood, and this allows us to examine a range of critical issues in a creative and resourceful way. A theory base is structured in each of the chapter themes, interspersed with leadership dimensions, issues, challenges and strategies. Wherever possible, current research and contemporary practices have been presented to extend the reader's understanding. A wide range of literature has been drawn on for each theme.

We have provided interviews and case studies with a range of early childhood colleagues to illustrate first-hand insight from a leadership perspective. We have deliberately provided material from Australia and from selected overseas countries. These national and international perspectives present the early childhood professional leader as a change agent, policy maker, advocate, quality assurance manager, conflict mediator, family- and futures-oriented administrator. Typically for the early childhood field, the reader will find many interchangeable terms used in this book, including child care, preschool, kindergarten, early years of school and children's services. These terms encompass the diverse contexts in which young children and their families interact with early childhood professionals. We invite readers to utilise the broad cross-cultural knowledge base presented in this book to explore the specific local contexts within their own communities in different and meaningful ways.

Outcomes are posed at the beginning of each chapter and are intended to help the reader focus on the particular theme and reflect on these as reading continues. Likewise, summaries at the end of chapters are designed to review the major issues presented.

Questions for reflection and discussion are posed at the end of each chapter. However, it is hoped that these questions are relevant for more than the one chapter theme and that readers will continue to analyse, critique and problem-solve in relation to the material presented by linking it to their own work or study situation. In doing this it is hoped that the reader will be futures-oriented and develop further insight into the role of a leader as a visionary, able to plan and articulate a strategic response to issues that emerge in their everyday work contexts.

Leadership is the dynamic and vibrant role expected of today's early childhood professionals. We do not believe that there are easy recipes to deal with the diverse contexts of contemporary early childhood settings. However, working effectively in multiethnic societies is both challenging and rewarding. Supportive, insightful partnerships with families and communities will continue to be a cornerstone of effective day-to-day practice. We hope that a range of readers, including students, early childhood and other human service providers, families and academics, will find the book helpful and inspiring.

Chapter 1

Administration, management and leadership: Connecting three key concepts in early childhood services

This chapter explores the three concepts of administration, management and leadership in relation to the early childhood field. It uses relevant theory and research to define and clarify the interconnections between these key concepts. It explains why it is necessary to deconstruct these concepts and evaluate their application in order to create new ways of thinking that are appropriate and relevant to contemporary practice. Evidence from relevant research is utilised to illuminate and support the overall approach adopted in this book.

Outcomes

At the conclusion of this chapter, the reader should have:

- developed an introductory understanding of three key concepts—administration, management and leadership— operationalised within early childhood contexts;

- a heightened awareness of some theoretical perspectives on administration, management and leadership;

- the skills to present selected relevant research on leadership;

- developed a framework through which to examine relationships across administration, management and leadership in early childhood.

CHILDREN'S SERVICES AS HUMAN SERVICES ORGANISATIONS

Preschools and childcare centres exist to support families with young children, and may be described as human services organisations (Hasenfeld 1983). Basically, this means that children's services are concerned with people. Human services can be:

> ... distinguished from other bureaucracies by two key characteristics. First, they work with and on people whose attributes they attempt to shape. People are in a sense their 'raw material'. Second, they are mandated—and thus justify their existence—to protect and promote the welfare of the people they serve.   (Hasenfeld 1983: 1).

As human services organisations, children's services are unique because of who they serve, the goals they aim to meet, and the way they are managed and administered. Labels such as family day care, long-day care, occasional care, preschools and school-age care reflect the range of services that may be defined as children's services. The type of services provided by each organisation varies according to factors such as the children's age, location and hours of availability. Each service may describe its goals in terms of education, care, welfare and the recreational needs of children and families. The overall philosophy and the nature of day-to-day operations are established depending on whether they are a private or public institution.

In most countries, there is a distinction made between children's services that are run by private entrepreneurs and those which are operated by non-commercial entities, such as charities, churches or community groups. In Australia, for instance, '73 per cent of centre based child care is provided by the private sector', and three levels of government deal with funding and policy responsibilities (Press & Hayes 2000: 21–5). These organisational factors have implications not only for those families for whom the service is directed but also for the staff employed to deliver the services. We develop propositions throughout this chapter which demonstrate:

- that there are interconnections between administration, management and leadership and that it is useful to clarify these connections;
- that early childhood centres are administratively complex and suffer from poor community perceptions of their role and image;
- that efficient administration of early childhood centres is dependent on clearly defined procedures and lines of responsibility;
- that exploration of the specific roles and responsibilities of the early childhood professional is a prerequisite to understanding leadership;
- that the early childhood leader's role is diffuse and poorly understood by the profession and wider community;

- that defining, understanding and applying sound leadership to early childhood contexts is fundamental to sound management;
- that obstacles to sound management including leadership can be identified and overcome;
- that skills, roles, responsibilities and dispositions are not mutually exclusive in administration, management and leadership;
- that new directions in leadership can be identified and applied; and
- that one can apply a framework of administration, management and leadership in order to clarify positions and ways forward.

Clients' satisfaction with early childhood services takes on a special significance through being a service directed at families with young children (Vining 1994). There is no agreement within the early childhood field as to who the primary client is: is it the child or the parents or both? Instead of disintegrating this dialogue into unproductive sectional interests, it is advisable to consider client satisfaction by focusing on the child within the context of the family. The task of finding out clients' needs and their degree of satisfaction with service delivery is indeed complex. The expert model of early childhood has promoted the image of an all-knowing early childhood professional (Stonehouse & Woodrow 1992: 208), as distinct from the parent, who has a limited understanding of early childhood matters. While early childhood professionals may have sound child-observation and program-planning skills, much of the child's background information needs to be obtained from the family or the guardians. Therefore, early childhood professionals' awareness and understanding of parents' knowledge as well as their aspirations and expectations for their children are fundamental in providing quality services.

Today, in many countries, various resource materials have been produced to help parents make decisions about their childcare choices. Newspaper articles, pamphlets and brochures contain information and questions that parents can ask staff when visiting a childcare centre or a preschool. Consider the following questions, which have been developed by the National Childcare Accreditation Council (NCAC) of Australia:

Choosing quality child care—questions to ask

- Are parents encouraged to participate in activities?
- Are families informed about proposed changes to policies?
- Is there a planned program of day-to-day activities for my child?
- Are individual learning goals set for my child?
- Are mealtimes pleasant?
- Do toileting, nappy-changing and rest times meet my child's individual needs?

- Are there activities to foster my child's creativity?
- Are there clear procedures for raising any concerns I may have?

(Adapted from NCAC 2001a: 2)

In the absence of published research, it is difficult to know exactly how parents use questions such as these: for example, do parents make decisions based on what they observed while visiting centres or do they question staff and/or other family and friends with experience in using children's services? To assess the usefulness of such promotional materials in selecting children's services, particularly in times of high demand and low supply, is also problematical. Nevertheless, it is worth considering the extent to which early childhood professionals are willing and are able to answer such questions, particularly in their initial interactions with families. An atmosphere of willingness to inform, share and work collaboratively with families needs to be established from the start, and such issues will be explored further in Chapter 3.

PERCEPTIONS AND PUBLIC IMAGE

Quentin Bryce, the inaugural Chief Executive Officer of the National Childcare Accreditation Council of Australia, stated that 'there is no task, no endeavour, no profession and no vocation more critical and more vital to our society than the care and education of children' (in Loane 1997: 287). Ironically, in the same book Sally Loane, the journalist who interviewed Bryce, concludes the chapter by stating that:

> It's a mystery and our shame. The fact that we do our best to keep these (early childhood) workers in the 'pink ghetto' says more than anything about how we, as a society, treat our children   (Loane 1997: 316).

An examination of how children's services have evolved in Western societies around the world shows that the development of children's services has been inextricably linked to the social structure and position of women in society (e.g. see Brennan 1998a and b; Hayden 2000; Petrie 1992). As a consequence, the status of early childhood workers as professionals is also tied up with gender and the cultural context of any given society. Based on the work of people such as Loane (1997), Rosier and Lloyd-Smith (1996) and Sumsion (2002), characteristics of early childhood professionals within the Australian context emerge as follows:

- underpaid—tertiary trained but low rates of pay for long hours of work;

- undervalued—perceived as an extension of women's nurturing role and domestic work as mothers in particular;
- poorly unionised—isolated small work units; diversity of unions and poor understanding of industrial rights;
- exploited—coerced into accepting variations to work conditions 'for the sake of the children'; and
- burnout and high rates of staff turnover—stressful and physically demanding work.

Having undertaken a study of television and video programs containing references to the use of formal child care, Hayden (1994: 14–15), for instance, concluded that 'the predominant image of child care perpetuates a myth that non-familial care is unnecessary at best and is dangerous at worst'. Such views ignore the fact that many governments, including Australia's, have taken on the responsibility of funding children's services as an avenue of infrastructure support to industry and businesses, to enable workers with family responsibilities for young children to participate in paid employment. Such a policy approach may also be conceived, in part, as an acknowledgment that children are a community concern. The extent to which governments fund and resource access to children's services of course varies significantly across countries, reflective of prevailing political ideologies as well as particular societal values and beliefs about children and women (Brennan 1998a; Press 1999; Zigler, Kagan & Hall 1996).

The early childhood profession is regarded as a 'pink ghetto', as it is a predominantly female occupation. The ideology of motherhood and the caretaking archetype (Robertson & Talley 2002: 10), perceived as an extension of the woman's role in the family context, is reinforced from within and without the profession (Keary 2000; Loane 1997; Petrie 1992) and has been a perpetual theme in writing about early childhood professionals. Reflecting over generational changes, Keary (2000: 17) concluded that:

> *Indeed it cannot be disputed that there is a plethora of fresh and diverse understandings and versions of mother/mothering. Perhaps the challenge for early childhood educators in the 21st century involves how to negotiate the possible conflicting views between, for example, working mothers and community mothers who care for their children; and how to encounter the ever changing anxieties, desires, needs, material conditions, and inequities attached to representations of mother/mothering.*

ROLES AND RESPONSIBILITIES

Medical practitioners perform tasks related to people's health and wellbeing and do not advise you about accountancy or how to complete your tax return.

Secondary school physics teachers do not front up to students doing their high school examinations and start teaching them history. But the early childhood professional is expected to perform a multitude of functions, and to be all things to all people. Employment of social workers in early childhood positions in government to deal with child protection matters is rarely questioned, but early childhood professionals do not seem to be able to take over jobs in the same way that social workers do. Why is this the case? Why is the early childhood profession then so vulnerable to takeover bids from other professions in the human services area? What do early childhood professionals need to do to replace our poor professional image with something more appropriate and reflective of the multiple roles we play?

The roles and responsibilities of professionals in early childhood have been defined and described in different ways by various authors in Australia and overseas. These include Australians such as Margaret Clyde, Jillian Rodd, Marjory Ebbeck and Anne Stonehouse and Americans such as Paula Jorde-Bloom, Sharon Lyn Kagan and Lillian Katz. In reviewing this literature, one must be clear first about what we mean by roles and responsibilities, and second about characteristics or elements that are peculiar to the early childhood field.

Roles and responsibilities:

- may be described and defined as activities and relationships expected of a person occupying a specific position;
- refer to a bundle of norms or commonly expected behaviours and sanctions that are expected of a person holding a particular position; this is called the 'role set';
- can be differentiated by
  - class—economic rewards and deprivation
  - status—prestige/esteem of the role
  - power—extent to which one is able to make decisions that affect others;
- are separated by time and space, and the individual can choose the role set to be expressed in a particular context;
- may not always be complementary or compatible, and 'role conflict' occurs when there is no match between the role set and the actual behaviour expressed by the individual.

Exploration of the specific roles and responsibilities of early childhood professionals is a prerequisite to studying leadership development. As Jalongo and Isenberg (2000: xxii) have commented, the beginning early childhood professional in particular has a rather idealised, romantic view of what it would be like to work with young children. They urge students:

... to get a realistic perspective of the realities of child care and education from the start. Otherwise, they feel disillusioned and defeated and leave the profession to which they were committed and for which they have been trained ...   (Jalongo & Isenberg 2000: xxiv)

There is much debate about whether or not there is a specific body of knowledge that is exclusive to the field of early childhood. Some people would argue that the roles and responsibilities of early childhood professionals have become so diffused that we can no longer see early childhood as a specialist field. Others believe that we have a specialist field of knowledge and that we should do everything possible to enhance it and advance it. The study of roles and responsibilities in early childhood has shifted the focus from teachers' personal characteristics to teacher performance and, more recently, to the study of thought processes, looking at teachers' beliefs and the values that guide their decision-making.

There is now a plethora of definitions and descriptions of the nature of work undertaken by early childhood professionals. Look at the descriptions in Figure 1.1, taken from four texts written during the 1970s and 80s by authors who were pioneers in writing about administration and management in early childhood. These four examples illustrate the diversity of roles and responsibilities expected of early childhood professionals. The wide-ranging expectations are indeed breathtaking, as they go well beyond the traditional teacher

Figure 1.1 What do early childhood professionals do? What do the experts say?

Almy (1975)
Parent educator; consultant; trainer; supervisor; code-enforcer; negotiator; institution builder; stage-setter; provisioner; researcher.

Decker and Decker (1984)
Service planner and evaluator; business affairs conductor; personnel services manager; supervisor and coordinator of maintenance; food service and transport; provider of channels of communication and information exchange.

Jorde-Bloom (1982)
Teacher; nurse; accountant; planner; counsellor; gardener; nutritionist; plumber; receptionist; fundraiser; artist; public relations expert; board member; children's advocate.

Sciarra and Dorsey (1979)
Goal-setter; teacher; administrator; financial manager; curriculum developer; lobbyist; parent and community liaison officer; trouble-shooter; advocate; cleaner; career information sharer.

Adapted from Simons (1986: 44).

responsibilities to include tasks dealing not only with service delivery, such as being a service planner and evaluator (Decker & Decker 1984: 169–70), but also with being a maintenance person, such as a gardener and a plumber (Jorde-Bloom 1982: 32). By reflecting on the similarities and differences of these descriptors, one could further consider:

- Do these authors use any common terms, and how have they evolved over time?
- Are there any terms that are no longer valid in today's world of work?
- What do these descriptions reflect about the early childhood profession?

Given the dominance and reliance on texts emanating from North America, for instance, readers may wish also to consider the cross-cultural transferability of such definitions.

Competencies of early childhood managers

While there may be little or no agreement about early childhood professionals' job descriptions, there is consensus that the current context of work is complex and is complicated by the rapid pace of societal change (e.g. see Hujala & Puriola 1998; Jalongo & Isenberg 2000). Depending on the service or the specific position, some roles are more necessary than others; depending on the person or the individual, some roles will be executed or implemented better or worse than others.

These traditional roles may be described as being relatively autonomous and self-contained, and early childhood professionals are popularly defined as 'teachers of young children' (e.g. see Almy 1975; Katz 1995). Some may question whether the term 'teacher' is appropriate and relevant, and others are concerned that the commonsense usage of the term 'teacher' may be damaging to the status of the profession. Such debates reinforce the fact that the contemporary roles of early childhood professionals are poorly defined, and do not necessarily cover the totality of the responsibilities involved in dealing with the child within the context of the family and society. Attempting to capture the spirit of this growing complexity, writers such as Hayden (1996) and Jorde-Bloom (1997) have adapted Sergiovanni's 'hierarchy of management forces' (1984) to take account of the particular characteristics of the early childhood field. Depicted originally as a pyramid, for ease of reading the competencies (i.e. roles and responsibilities) are listed in Figure 1.2 under each level in a stepwise fashion, with arrows showing upward movement from the technical to the cultural and symbolic competencies.

Figure 1.2 Hierarchy of competencies for early childhood managers

Level 5: **Cultural and symbolic functions**

Public presentations, political campaigning, use of the media; articulating a vision and promoting a collective identity for all

Level 4: **Public relations functions**

Community outreach and advocacy, networking, dealing with government and non-government agencies, fundraising, marketing and planning special events

Level 3: **Client-oriented functions**

Dealing with children and families, curriculum development, overseeing the implementation of Developmentally Appropriate Practices (DAP) to ensure high-quality service delivery, assessment and making referrals

Level 2: **Staffing functions**

Related to interpersonal aspects including supervision, mentoring, performance appraisal, team building, resolving staff conflict, professional development and creating a positive organisational climate

Level 1: **Technical functions**

Related to keeping the centre in operation, including purchasing, budgeting, record-keeping, hiring and firing staff, doing rosters, developing policies and writing reports

Adapted from Hayden (1996) and Jorde-Bloom (1997).

Figure 1.2 illustrates generic roles and responsibilities of centre directors and is therefore centre-specific and position-specific. This model does not necessarily reflect the diversity of the early childhood professionals' work environments, especially those in family day care and policy advisory positions in government departments. Nor does it represent the variety of functions carried out by other centre-based early childhood professionals, such as teachers and childcare assistants.

At each level of achievement, growing in competence, the early childhood professional moves on and away from the centre and into the public arena. Hayden (1996) says that, to be a good manager, one has first to be able to perform the technical tasks that are placed at the base of the hierarchy. Only then can one focus on the staffing aspects, including mentoring and inspiring staff, and building a team-based work environment. Staff need to feel as if the director cares, listens, and helps when needed. The next thing is to ensure a sound basis of program development. Jorde-Bloom (1997: 36) writes that just because one is a good teacher, it does not mean that one can manage the overall centre. Holding together diverse views that subscribe to a common philosophy is not easily done. It is only when the centre's philosophy and policies are in place that the early childhood professional should move out into the public arena, and this includes responsibilities outside the centre. There is no point in promoting the importance of high-quality standards unless a centre can demonstrate this through the program and services provided.

One of the main strengths of this model is that it takes into account multiple roles performed by contemporary early childhood professionals. There is also progress from one level to the next. Given that career advancement within early childhood is unclear, this type of progression is important because it gives hope and direction, based on a strategic planning approach. The model is goal-directed and achievable, irrespective of the mandatory or elective nature of roles and responsibilities performed by early childhood professionals in the director's position. Accordingly, this model could be used as a practical tool in determining performance targets, especially in terms of centre administration and management.

ADMINISTRATION, MANAGEMENT AND LEADERSHIP: MAKING THE CONNECTIONS

Administration, management and leadership are three concepts that are often used interchangeably by authors, even when each one means something completely different. There is little or no consensus among scholars, researchers or practitioners working in either early childhood or business studies and accounting about the best way to define these terms. In this book we want to explore the interconnections between administration, management and leadership in an integrated way. We will begin the process by attempting to deconstruct the three concepts and thereby demonstrate the complexities and subtleties involved in implementing tasks considered to be in this domain. In order to provide some coherence to understanding the organisational contexts of early childhood services today, we provide an overarching framework that brings together the various dispositions, skills and roles related to administration, management and leadership.

Using the analogy of a house, administration may be described as the 'supporting beams of a building' or the 'supporting framework that holds the centre together' (Jorde-Bloom, Sheerer & Britz 1991a: 11). Administrative functions usually refer directly to the policies and procedures that are put in place to run the centre's daily operations. Sometimes they are described as the 'housekeeping tasks', and reflect the lower status accorded to administrative roles and responsibilities. This is not an uncommon perception within the early childhood profession itself. It is thought that administrative tasks can be carried out by anyone, and that one does not require specific training in early childhood to learn about centre administration.

A quarter of a century ago, the famous early educator Millie Almy (1975: 143) described administration as 'the stage setting or facilitative functions acknowledging that carrying out administrative functions' requires early childhood professionals to step outside and go beyond their educative roles and responsibilities. There is an emerging consensus on this view, as explained by Hayden (1996: 2), who claimed that to become effective managers of a child care centre early childhood professionals require a different set of skills that:

> . . . have little bearing upon the teaching function. Administrators need skills in planning and organisational development, management of physical and human resources, team building, working with diverse groups of adults, complex financial accounting, communication at all levels, report writing, liaison and other public relations functions, amongst others.

In essence, administration is only *one* component or dimension of management, which contains the overall processes of centre coordination, including decision-making, communication and problem-solving processes. Leadership, in turn, is an extension of management, concerned more with the long-term objectives, including the articulation and development of the centre's vision for the future.

Leadership 'is more than routine management which focuses on the present and is dominated by issues of continuity and stability' (Simons 1986, in Rodd 1996: 4). By putting in place policies and procedures it is hoped that there will be consistency and equity of treatment for all concerned—parents, staff and children. The resultant sense of security augurs well in promoting organisational stability. Rodd (1996: 5) suggests that:

> . . . a person with highly developed management skills is likely to have structured the administration of the program to give herself adequate time to devote to key leadership functions. A person with poorly developed management skills is

unlikely to be sufficiently organised to free up the time needed to focus upon lead-
ership issues.

Accordingly, Rodd (1996: 5) concluded that 'successful leaders are more than efficient managers', and therefore 'management skills are necessary but not sufficient for effective leadership'. This view was strongly supported by research undertaken by Waniganayake, Morda and Kapsalakis (2000: 15), who found that:

> *. . . personal attributes and/or skills beyond the responsibilities of centre man-*
> *agement (such as adaptability, awareness and active involvement in leading the*
> *centre) were . . . critical competencies necessary to be recognized as a leader.*

Organisational contexts of leadership

All children's centres and/or programs require some form of administration, management and leadership. The size of the centre/program, its owner/ sponsor and its program objectives may define the nature and type of systems set up to guide these functions. For instance, infant and toddler programs require different space and equipment from those of preschools. Similarly, centres relying on government funds may differ from those that are linked to workplaces such as banks, hospitals and universities. Referring to the comments of a teacher describing the nature of administration in her school, Almy (1975) alerts us to be cautious about becoming 'compartmentalized' by setting up administrative structures and systems which are overly bureaucratic and rigidly rule-governed:

> *Life in school is carefully compartmentalized. There is the box of the classroom*
> *with its smaller boxes for gym and cluster teachers and library. There is the box of*
> *staff relations, with small boxes inside for different grades and groupings. There*
> *are the authority boxes, supervisory and union, and it is becoming increasingly dif-*
> *ficult to tell them apart. There are the boxes of relations with custodians, school*
> *aides, and para-professionals, parents, community people and other such lesser*
> *forms of life   (Almy 1975: 16)*

This illustration is a timely reminder to early childhood professionals not to forget the big picture at the expense of the minutiae. Given the rapidity of change being forced on organisational contexts such as children's services, it is essential that whatever systems of administration and management are established, they can be flexible and adaptable in meeting the needs of the service users. In responding to change, children and families as well as the service providers (i.e. staff) must be satisfied that there has been minimal interference with service quality.

It is also important to note that the particular functions of administration, management and leadership may not be restricted to one or two specific individuals within the centre. While the centre director, for example, may have the major responsibility for overseeing the development of the centre's budget, s/he will require input from all staff regarding various financial aspects, such as what equipment to buy and the special needs of particular children. Similarly, in implementing the curriculum all teaching staff must carry out a number of regular administrative tasks, such as observing and recording children's developmental progress and preparing a weekly or monthly schedule of learning activities for each group of children. Together, all staff as a team must plan, implement and evaluate the centre's programs and services. Accordingly, administrative tasks are often a shared responsibility, requiring cooperation at different levels throughout the centre.

Working with others, by sharing your skills and experiences as well as accommodating the expertise of others at the centre, ensures the successful operation of the centre. This involves following set administrative policies and procedures, specific to each centre/program. However, such policies will not always be written down (i.e. formal). Some procedures are considered 'custom and practice' (i.e. informal). 'That's how we've always done it!' is a popular phrase used by those who defer to informal policies and procedures to explain their actions. The implications of not having written policies and procedures are considered in Chapter 5.

Impact of organisational structures

Despite the kaleidoscopic variation of children's services found in any one country, there are some common core structures found in most early childhood organisations (Decker & Decker 1988: 169). One of these is the establishment of the position of centre director or coordinator, who is responsible for the day-to-day operation of the centre. Making sure that the centre is open and running effectively each day is at the heart of the director's general responsibilities. The actual duties and tasks performed by the director, however, will vary significantly due to a number of factors, including the following:

- ## The size of the centre

  Depending on the number of children enrolled and allowed under local regulations, a centre could be administered by a single person or a group of staff. Within a small group of staff, smaller than 10 for instance, the degree of specialisation and delegation is limited; the extent of collaboration here may be more intense and necessary, as the centre relies on all staff working together.

- ### *The ages of the children using the centre*

    Government regulations tend to differentiate staffing requirements according to age cohorts, as per infants, toddlers, preschoolers, or a combination of any of these categories. Staffing levels in turn are linked to children's ages as well as the numbers in a group.

- ### *Who the centre owner/proprietor or sponsor is*

    Children's services may be delivered by a church-based organisation (e.g. a non-profit preschool), a hospital (e.g. a work-based childcare centre), a school (e.g. an after-school-care program) or a local municipal authority (e.g. a family day care service). Centres may be a private enterprise owned by an individual or managed under a franchise or chain. The contractual arrangements under which the centre's licence was obtained have a direct link with who administers it and what types of structures and processes are put in place to organise service delivery.

Each centre is unique, and the lines of authority for administration and management will depend on the type of structures that are in place. Efficient administration of a centre is based on having clearly defined procedures and domains of responsibility. The authority and responsibility allocated to specific positions determine the lines of communication and decision making within an organisation. The extent of centralisation and decentralisation will vary between organisations, as will the nature of tasks that have to be completed (Hildebrand & Hearron 1997: 100).

Taken together, the major operational tasks that are common and necessary to ensure the smooth and efficient functioning of an early childhood centre include the following:

- financial administration;
- maintenance of records for personnel, property and services;
- compliance with all regulatory requirements; and
- centre evaluation.

A similar approach is adopted by Broinowski (1994: 2), who refers to childcare centre administration as 'management practice' or 'the practical application of management theories'. According to him, establishment of an efficient information system is central to effective administration. In carrying out administrative functions, staff need to have a sound understanding of several key concepts, such as confidentiality, accountability, evaluation and compliance. A brief discussion of these concepts is presented next.

Confidentiality

Confidentiality is about trust and reliability, an assurance that privacy will be protected. Issues of confidentiality cut across all matters of administration, management and leadership in children's services. When taking observations of children's growth and development, when evaluating program plans or writing reports on accidents and injuries at the centre, staff must be vigilant about remaining objective and non-judgmental. Various staff as well as parents may access these documents. For the protection of individual privacy, there has to be clear policy regarding lines of authority and responsibility in handling information, especially those records and reports deemed confidential by parents. Early childhood professionals need to be aware of the consequences of giving out the simplest piece of information pertaining to a child, a family or the centre to another person. For example, before disclosing the home contact details of a child's friend to send a birthday invitation, one must get parents' permission first. The procedure early childhood professionals should follow in disclosing information to other families or professionals may not always be clear. The onus is on the centre and the staff to be aware and informed of the extent of liability—legal (refer to state privacy laws for instance) as well as professional and moral (e.g. the Code of Professional Conduct). One must seek advice early and be prepared by reviewing existing policies and procedures of the centre to ensure confidentiality for all—children, parents and staff.

Accountability

Over the years, the focus of government funding has shifted from evaluation to accountability. The limitations of summative evaluations, particularly in relation to difficulties associated with isolating specific goals and reliable indicators demonstrating the achievement of goals, are now well recognised. Yet attempts to measure achievements in monetary terms or via performance indicators equated with monetary value can place severe restrictions on community programs such as children's services. Fiscal accountability is achievable through bureaucratic processes. However, increased bureaucracy (or paperwork) is usually an indicator of reduced face-to-face contact with clients and employees (Ebbeck & Ebbeck 1994: 18).

When providing services to clients as well as receiving government funding, an organisation (or an individual) is obliged to meet certain requirements to ensure that the services are delivered in an efficient and effective manner. This is the way in which the organisation and/or the individual who is also the licensee of a centre remain accountable to clients as well as to the sponsor of the service. In discussing the importance of accountability in early childhood, Ebbeck and Ebbeck (1994: 20) concluded that:

It is desirable to view accountability as a reciprocal rather than a hierarchical arrangement. Likewise, a comprehensive rather than a narrow approach to accountability is more applicable to the early childhood field.

Evaluation

State regulatory authorities usually require children's services to set in place policies and procedures to monitor service quality. The licensing standards are the basic minimum requirements, but to achieve a higher standard of quality service delivery a variety of procedures must be in place. Hildebrand and Hearron (1997: 193) state: 'monitoring and controlling for quality are functions that each staff member must be concerned about daily, hourly, and moment to moment'. Some of these instruments and systems of quality assessment and improvement may be externally controlled, such as in the case of the National Childcare Accreditation Council's principles, used to accredit childcare centres and family day care schemes in Australia. These principles require services to adhere to quality standards beyond the licensing requirements, and are discussed further in Chapter 4.

Compliance

To comply is to act according to set rules or directives. With reference to children's services, the notion of compliance means acting in accordance with or in keeping with the requirements set out by various authorities linked to the centre's operation. The types of compliance enforced by the various authorities will differ according to the type of services provided and the centre's management structure. The most common form of compliance is linked to the government department responsible for licensing children's services. Compliance with these regulations is usually compulsory, and failure to follow these, or 'non-compliance', can result in penalties, fines or deregistration.

Departmental officers who are employed to monitor the implementation of children's services regulations may have wide-ranging powers under legislation. It is possible, for example, that leaving the rubbish bins without a lid will be regarded as a mere technical breach, while staff yelling at children is a serious offence. Puddles of water in the corridor or leaving food rotting in the fridge can be hazardous to the health and safety of both children and staff. One of these matters by itself may not be regarded as a major offence or a non-compliance indicator requiring a severe penalty. However, the centre may be put on notice and revisited more often before reregistration is granted. The level of 'seriousness' may or may not be clarified in the legislative documents, and is best explained by the local enforcement authorities. The onus is on the centre staff and management to ensure that services are provided in accordance with local laws and regulations. To comply in a legal sense is a technical requirement. Leadership is necessary to ensure that the intent and the spirit of the law are upheld from a values perspective.

DEFINITIONS AND DISCOURSE IN LEADERSHIP

Currently, there is no agreed definition of leadership in the early childhood field, nor do we have a publicly acknowledged list of our leaders and of what we expect of our leaders. During the early 1990s, a group of academics from Finland, England, Australia, the USA and Russia established the International Leadership Project (ILP) to explore the conceptualisation of leadership in early childhood in their countries. The leadership model of the ILP was contextually located within an ecological framework, where children, parents and early childhood personnel were organised as a broader social system. It was proposed that leadership arises through interactions between actors and structures within differing organisational settings. The challenge was to ascertain the nature and significance of early childhood leadership as well as to explore the roles and responsibilities attached to leadership within diverse societal contexts.

The background of the ILP is documented in Hujala and Puroila (1998), and papers published subsequently discuss more specific findings. Waniganayake and Hujala (2001), for instance, discuss the way in which participants from Finland identified workers such as Frobel and Piaget as leaders in early childhood. In contrast, Australian participants identified over 50 local women, including academics and civil servants, who were central to the development of the early childhood field nationally. This study highlighted the differing perceptions of leadership, reflecting the impact of cultural and historical forces on the evolution of the profession in the two countries. Indeed, the only similarity between Finland and Australia was that the majority of those people listed as 'leaders' were no longer alive. The extent to which longevity influenced status and recognition of leadership was, however, not assessed in the ILP study. In this regard, Kagan's comments are salutary:

> Indeed so weighty are the expectations for leaders as individuals—and for leadership as a concept—that some suggest that it has been romanticised beyond reality, likened to penicillin as a quick, one-shot cure-all for social and organisational ills.   (Kagan 1994: 50)

Undoubtedly, leadership is one of the most critical concepts or phenomena under discussion in the early childhood field today, and this interest in leadership matters is relatively new (Rodd 1994, 1998). Traditionally, leadership studies have been linked to business studies as a skill or component related to administration and management. During the 1990s, the inappropriateness of this approach was highlighted by those such as Mitchell (1990: 1), who lamented that, in spite of this understanding, 'new theories of leadership are more concerned with what leaders do than what leadership is'. Nivala (1998) added that research-based theory development in leadership studies has a brief and short history, and the extent to which we can describe existing models of leadership as 'theories' is questionable. Adopting a similar approach to that taken by writers such as Sciarra & Dorsey (2000: 6), leadership notions can be further explored by considering a selected range of contemporary definitions, as presented below.

Ways of defining leadership

- 'Leadership is a set of reciprocal relationships, not a static quality' (Morgan 1997: 13).
- 'Leadership is the ability to influence others, especially in getting others to reach challenging goals' (Chapman & O'Neil 2000: 2).
- Leadership is 'is a fragile commodity, earned over time. It can accrue to individuals and to organisations' (Kagan & Bowman 1997: xii).
- 'Leadership means both managing today and navigating the centre to the future' (Nivala 1998: 15).
- 'Leadership is . . . purposeful behaviour of influencing others to contribute to a commonly agreed goal for the benefit of individuals as well as the organisation or common good' (Sarros & Butchatsky 1996: 3).
- 'Leadership requires a positive sense of self, of knowing our boundaries and our linkages' (Cox 1996: 266).

From the above definitions it is clear that leadership is multifaceted and may be described in different ways. There is agreement among these authors that leadership grows through interaction with others, and the relationships that evolve between leaders and followers are crucial in sustaining leadership. In the same way, there are many ways of defining the essential skills and characteristics of leaders. According to Rodd (1998: 3), the five key elements of effective leadership are the leader's ability to:

1. provide a vision and communicate it;
2. develop a team culture;
3. set goals and objectives;
4. monitor and communicate achievements; and
5. facilitate and encourage the development of individuals.

These characteristics align leadership issues with centre-based activities in early childhood. This approach can narrow our focus on leadership to centre-based contexts, with the danger that leadership will be perceived as a positional status occupied usually by centre directors. Exploring this concern, in their research Waniganayake, Morda and Kapsalakis (2000) found that childcare centres do have the potential to promote leadership but that lack of real power in decision-making can contain leadership growth to hierarchical positions. As a way forward, it is argued that the roles and responsibilities of centre-based early childhood professionals 'need to be well defined to ensure purposeful activity, expanded to include more opportunities to lead, and legitimated so that task sharing can maximize wholesome centre operations' (Rosemary, Roskos, Owendorf & Olsen 1998: 202).

Figure 1.3 Leadership theories—key characteristics

---

1. Trait approaches

- Focus on characteristics and qualities of leaders
- Assumes that leaders are born, not made
- Aspects regularly identified with leaders include: intelligence, self-confidence, charisma, trustworthiness, decisiveness, ability to communicate well, and high energy levels
- Limited application: doesn't take into account followers and the situational context
- Highly personalised, subjective view of leadership

---

2. Behavioural approaches

- Focus on leadership functions and style; the ways in which leaders approach work
- Functions relate to (i) tasks or problems and (ii) group maintenance or social aspects
- Leadership style reflects a task-centred or group-centred approach
- Separates leadership from management

management = process
versus
leadership = product

---

3. Contingency approaches

- Focus on the situation/circumstances; matches leadership to needs of a given situation
- Situational aspects include: organisational climate, nature of the tasks, pressure of time; attitudes of clients
- Leadership requires ongoing assessment and realignment to deal with changing demands of the organisation

---

The way in which various authors approach the study of leadership will of course reflect their particular field of interest and/or expertise. Broadly speaking, there are at least three perspectives on approaching the study of leadership, as indicated in Figure 1.3. None of these three approaches, by itself, provides a satisfactory explanation of the nature of leadership, its functions and significance in a particular organisational context. Perhaps more importantly, it must be emphasised that these traditional approaches do not present a cohesive and meaningful pathway towards understanding how leadership works within the early childhood field, and this requires some clarity.

Why do traditional leadership theories not work in early childhood?

As stated earlier, even though the study of leadership within the early childhood field is relatively new, there is an extensive body of literature on leadership theory in other disciplines, primarily in the business field (Nivala 1998; Sciarra & Dorsey 2000). There are some elements of the traditional leadership theories, such as the importance of vision, ethics and risk taking, which are relevant and applicable to early childhood. However, Kagan (1994: 51) argues that it is equally important to examine 'several critical assumptions which do not fully correspond with the nature of leadership in early education and care today'. These are as follows:

- *Assumption 1*

  That leadership is about a single person, usually a man, who holds the top position of an organisation such as Chief Executive Officer or President.

  Early childhood perspective: Staff are predominantly female and decision-making occurs on a collective or group basis involving parents and staff within each centre or service.

- *Assumption 2*

  That leaders are concerned with product-oriented, large organisations consisting of systems of rigid, formal, bureaucratic rules governing behaviour and hierarchical line management.

  Early childhood perspective: Smaller, more informal, and structurally more diffused organisations providing people-oriented services which are concerned with children and their families. Change is continuous, and therefore offers a more flexible, diverse and individualised approach to programs.

- *Assumption 3*

  That leadership is based on an ethos of competition (i.e. the focus is on rivalry and opposition); collaboration usually means corporate takeovers and mergers.

Early childhood perspective: Commitment to collaboration and coopera-tion (i.e. the focus is on 'working with others'). Competition is present but orientation or purpose of competition takes on a more just, humane, societal or community perspective.

Accordingly, Kagan (1994: 52) concluded that 'Traditional leadership theory is like the proverbial square peg that does not neatly fit the round hole of today's early childhood realities'. There are strong indicators that exploration of lead-ership in early childhood is continuing to engage researchers in countries such as Australia. For instance, the *Australian Journal of Early Childhood* published a special thematic edition on leadership in 2000, with five articles exploring new dimensions such as ethics and leadership, and health promotion as a new leadership function. Such publications offer new insight and will enhance the early childhood professional's struggle to reconceptualise, articulate and implement leadership in meaningful ways that are relevant for contemporary contexts in early childhood.

In a seminal text, Jillian Rodd (1994, 1998), one of Australia's pioneer researchers in leadership matters, provides a useful background to under-standing leadership in early childhood as a professional issue. In the follow-ing excerpt, Rodd discusses the challenges she encountered in conducting research into leadership in early childhood, and presents her current views on leadership matters, including advice to new graduates about the importance of leadership in early childhood.

Doing research on leadership

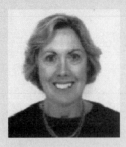

DR JILLIAN RODD
Early Childhood Consultant
United Kingdom

1. You are one of the pioneer researchers who realised the need to study lead-ership in early childhood. What were some of the challenges you encountered when conducting research into leadership in early childhood?

When I started examining leadership in early childhood, the biggest challenge I faced was practitioners' reluctance to identify themselves as leaders. My early research relied on information collected from a written questionnaire. However,

Continued

I found that I was not getting the information I was expecting so I changed the data-collection method from survey questionnaires to structured interviews. Data from the questionnaires and interviews with coordinators, teachers and childcare staff revealed that a significant percentage of participants did not perceive themselves to be in leadership roles, to undertake leadership responsibilities or to display leadership behaviour.

When I first approached people to participate in the research, a lot of them said 'I'm not a leader, I just manage/work in the centre'. They appeared not to understand what leadership was about, what was involved in being a leader or what aspects of their work were related to leadership. I had to ask people questions, such as 'Do you have a vision of where the centre is going in the future?', 'Do you have responsibility for organising and coordinating resources?', 'Do you work as a team member?', 'Do you plan, monitor and evaluate centre activity against goals and objectives?' etc. When the response was positive, I would point out how that response was related to leadership. A lot of participants then expressed amazement at how much of their day-to-day work was classified as leadership. Once people understood how leadership was displayed in their work, they were able to articulate considerable insight into aspects of leadership in early childhood centres. But helping people to understand initially that they were leaders who undertook leadership roles and responsibilities was the biggest hurdle to conducting an interview.

The other big challenge was time. People need time to prepare for an interview: to think about their work, what it involves and how they undertake it. In my research, I found that the best interviews were with people who had spent some time thinking about these issues before the formal research interview. It is very difficult for people to collect and articulate their thoughts about such a complex subject 'on the spot'. Therefore, I think that people need careful preparation and guidance in order to help them explain what leadership is and how it is displayed in early childhood centres. To do this well means that the researcher needs to talk to participants in order to ascertain their understanding about leadership and their work before conducting the formal interview. There are greater demands on the time of both researcher and participant in preparation for an interview that taps the deep understanding about issues related to leadership in early childhood.

2. In your opinion, is being a leader in early childhood different from being a leader in any other field?

Being a leader in early childhood is not at all different from being a leader in any other field. Effective leadership, be it of a large multinational company or a childcare centre, requires certain attitudes, attributes and skills. These include being an effective communicator and team builder, creating a motivating and rewarding work environment, and supporting the professional development of staff by ensuring they have access to appropriate support and training. Regardless of where they work or with whom they work, effective leaders bring out the best in their staff by respecting and valuing each person's unique combination of knowledge, skills and experience, by consulting and involving them in all aspects of running a centre, by keeping them informed about what is happening and what needs to happen to achieve the centre's vision and goals, by recognising

Continued

individual contributions and achievements and by delegating meaningful and important tasks in ways that enhance self-confidence and self-esteem in staff. This is what leadership is about in early childhood centres and why good leadership promotes quality practice.

3. What advice would you give to new graduates about the importance of leadership in early childhood?

Research evidence continues to support the strong relationship between leadership and quality in early childhood centres. Therefore, effective leadership is crucial for establishing and sustaining early childhood centres that are characterised by clear vision, strong professional values, recognised professional expertise and competence, high staff morale, committed and enthusiastic staff, positive, growing and supportive teams, and low staff turnover. Although the coordinator of a centre will assume significant leadership responsibility, leadership is not the sole responsibility of any one person. Everybody working in a centre can and should develop and exercise their leadership qualities and potential.

Effective leaders show concern and respect for their colleagues, empower them by encouraging involvement and ownership, support them in developing their strengths and achieving their aspirations and create a 'high challenge: low threat' working environment. Even in one's first job, leadership can be displayed by the way one communicates with others, works as a committed team member, accepts more challenging tasks and responsibilities, acts as a positive role model and mentor, and supports the professional development of others. Being technically proficient in working with young children and their parents is necessary but not sufficient to be an effective early childhood professional. Developing and displaying leadership is fundamental to and a crucial aspect of becoming an early childhood professional who ensures high-quality care and education for young children.

MENTORING AS A LEADERSHIP STRATEGY

Today, the term 'mentor' is being used everywhere by everybody. Being a 'mentor' and the process of 'mentoring' are 21st century buzzwords. However, one hopes that the noble art of mentoring does not travel down the commercial route of a fashion trend and lose its value, because mentoring someone is one of the most powerful means of effecting change. Mentoring is a concept built on relationships, and it is concerned with extending one's understanding and knowledge about working with others. Keeping in mind that humans are social creatures, learning how to relate to each other is fundamental for the survival of humankind. We also know that social skills have to be learnt, and mentoring, as a process, enables us to practise social skills in a variety of ways. Accordingly, mentoring goes to the heart of what it means to be a social being. As is shown in Figure 1.4, mentors can be described in a variety of ways.

Figure 1.4 Who or what is a mentor?

A mentor is . . .

- a trainer, developer, teacher, coach
- a supportive and more experienced colleague
- a confidant, counsellor and adviser
- a protector and a defender
- a source of information and knowledge

Taken together, the descriptors identified in Figure 1.4 denote the traditional meaning of a mentor. The concept of mentoring originated from Greek mythology, in which Ulysses entrusted the care of his young son Telemachus to his most loyal and trusted friend, Mentor. It was Mentor's responsibility to take care of the young boy when his father, Ulysses, was away on long trips defending the empire. Mentor's roles included being a guide, counsellor, tutor, coach, sponsor and defender of Telemachus, and dispensing discipline during his father's absence. The idea behind such an arrangement was that under Mentor's tutorage (i.e. being mentored) the protégé, Telemachus, would acquire the skills and knowledge to be a strong and effective citizen (Hays, Gerber & Minichiello 1999: 85; Rosenbach 1999).

One of the key outcomes of this type of traditional, one-to-one mentoring is that it facilitates the maintenance and continuation of a particular style of leadership. This is the downside of the traditional patriarchal model, because it is based on the command-and-follow approach to leadership: the mentor commands and the protégé follows. In effect, it is a classic example of cloning, where the protégé is expected to master and mirror the mentor. A collective model of mentoring, where a whole group is mentored, offers an alternative approach. The teaching and learning that occurs in the collective model of mentoring is more powerful because of the alliances that are built within a group of people with similar interests. Here the emphasis is on the process and not the person; on the relationships and not on the performance.

Mentoring is a strategic approach that can lead to rich rewards in the long term. The building of a learning community or a common culture within an organisation is an important outcome of collective mentoring. In such a community there is a commitment to learn and create new understandings and knowledge. In a learning organisation, through mentoring, it is possible to establish '. . . a holistic, yet individual and experiential approach to learning' (Hays, Gerber & Minichiello 1999: 86). This process can be seen as the establishment of critical mass—a powerful foundation, a stepping stone towards change. Rosenbach (1999: 5), who described mentoring as a 'a powerful force in leadership development', discusses the specific benefits of mentoring from the perspective of the protégé, the mentor and the organisation. This discussion is particularly helpful for those considering the establishment of formal mentoring systems in their organisations.

One must also take into account the limitations of mentoring, including dependency and discrimination, particularly in organisational contexts, as discussed by those such as Rosenbach (1999) and Hays, Gerber and Minichiello (1999). The degree of learning that can occur through mentoring can be measured by exploring changes in people's behaviour, attitudes and perceptions. Mentoring is also about values and ethics. The first step in developing a mentoring relationship is having credibility and gaining trust. These two ingredients are essential to creating a climate for change. The mentor and protégé must be clear about goals and their obligations to each other by staying in touch and communicating with each other openly and transparently (Kirner & Rayner 1999: 123). Figure 1.5 provides questions that early childhood professionals might consider when selecting a mentor.

Figure 1.5 Some questions to consider

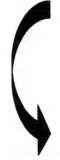

Selecting a mentor

- Is the mentor good at what s/he does?
- Is the mentor a good teacher as well as a good practitioner?
- Can the mentor motivate/inspire?
- What needs and goals do you both want to pursue through this mentorship?
- What is the mentor's status/position within the organisation/profession?
- What is the chemistry and rapport between the participants?
- Is the mentor flexible and available, especially when most needed?

If you were the mentor, how would YOU respond to these questions?

Adapted from Zey (1995).

Not all questions will be relevant or meaningful for everyone. For instance, if one is seeking a mentor within the same organisation, there are separate issues to consider, such as what impact positional responsibilities and authority structures may have on the mentoring relationship. Some of these considerations are explored by Christine Chen, the founding President of the Association for Early Childhood Educators in Singapore (AECES). In the following excerpt she discusses her perspectives and experiences about mentoring. In particular, Dr Chen's comments reflect a national or cultural influence in the way a person selects another person as a suitable mentor.

Perspectives on mentoring

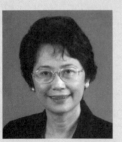

DR CHRISTINE CHEN
President
Association for Early Childhood Educators in Singapore
(AECES)
Singapore

1. As early childhood practitioners, does it matter if your mentor has expertise in early childhood, or could it be someone from another discipline or work experience?

In my research, most of the mentees, when they referred to their mentors, never spoke about their area of expertise. Mentees needed to feel comfortable with the mentor and they needed to be able to relate to the mentor personally. From the mentors' perspective, their role was just 'giving my two cents worth', acting as a 'safety net' or 'safety belt'. Therefore, having expert knowledge has never been an issue. As such, I don't think having expert knowledge in early childhood is the critical issue. Personally, I have a mentee who now works in human resource development; I was his social work field adviser when he was a student. He still calls me up once in a while for career options and what he should do with his 2-year-old daughter. Mentoring is about guiding someone through life's journey.

2. Can your boss be your mentor?

Speaking from my personal experience, I found I was able to mentor all my teachers who were working in the centre I was directing. I have individual conferences with my teachers three to four times a year, of which one will be to give a rise in salary. Every time I have to ask the teacher how much she makes, I apologise for my ignorance and tell my teachers that I can never remember individual staff salaries. Once one of them replied (her statement still rings in my mind): 'But Mrs Chen, you will always remember what happens to my daughter, my husband ...!'. Like I said, mentees look for that personal element in the mentor, and if the boss can relate to the mentee at a personal level a mentoring relationship develops. Mentoring is about guiding someone, and your boss can mentor you about career options.

3. I am aware that you have established a system of leadership mentoring through the Association for Early Childhood Educators in Singapore. Could you please describe this and what you have been able to achieve through this to date?

I am STILL TRYING to install the system. My model is to have AECES tutors go through mentoring workshops, and then have them 'hand-hold' directors and

Continued

have the directors hand-hold the teachers. So far, the AECES tutors have gone through the mentor workshop and I am planning workshops for AECES members who are directors or teachers. The problem we are facing is that everyone is so busy, and we cannot find a date to carry out these workshops. After the mentoring workshops AECES will place students training to become early childhood professionals with these mentors. Based on feedback on how the mentors are able to guide these students, they will be issued a certificate. These evaluation and feedback mechanisms are currently being developed.

OBSTACLES TO LEADERSHIP DEVELOPMENT IN EARLY CHILDHOOD

By looking at developments in the USA, Morgan (1997) discusses the roots of early childhood leadership in her country. Reading her comments in conjunction with Kagan and Bowman (1997: 3–8) and Rodd (1998: 1–30) provides sufficient information for an understanding of the broader historical context of early childhood leadership. It shows that leadership development within the early childhood field has been inhibited by factors within and without, and these include the following:

- *Lack of an agreed definition of leadership and an accepted list of characteristics of a leader in early childhood* (as discussed earlier in this chapter).
- *Ambivalence about authority.* Many early childhood professionals do not want to engage in discussions about power and authority, seeing both as being outside their professional responsibilities in working with children and their families. In this sense leadership is seen as something to do with power, a takeover, and is associated with aggression. It is therefore not something that early childhood professionals, who are 'nice ladies', ought to be concerned with. Such a view highlights misunderstandings arising out of a view that all authority is about a single person's power.
- *Lack of systems thinking.* This is reflected in the early childhood professional's inability to adopt an integrated and holistic perspective and the desire to break everything down into its components. So when we talk about the child we talk of social, emotional, physical and cognitive development and then say very little about the child within the context of the family and society. Accordingly we need a multidimensional perspective, not a narrow programmatic approach, to the study of leadership.
- *Scarce resources and inappropriate competition.* Some competition is healthy—for example, when linking policy development in health care for the young and the old. However, due to limited resources, instead

of linking generational planning we tend to divide scarce resources, usually on the basis of administrators' perceptions of competing demands.

- *Narrow preparation for leadership roles and responsibilities through pre-service training programs.* By and large, early childhood professionals' values are connected with serving children (Hujala & Puroila 1998), and they do not trust those concerned with equating money with service. This, too, is a rather narrow view of the work performed by contemporary early childhood professionals.
- *Poor public perceptions of women in leadership positions.* One major consequence is that 'by judging ourselves and other women by rules we haven't had a say in making, leaders act as agents of social control to restrict the activities of women' (Cox 1996: 13).

Constraints on leadership development in early childhood are addressed in more detail in Kagan and Bowman (1997). In this book various authors explore challenges faced by early childhood leaders in terms of institutional and racial bias, lack of recognition and remuneration, poor training and service delivery as well as personal attributes of leaders, such as ambivalence towards power and authority. Having acknowledged these barriers to leadership growth in early childhood, it is now imperative we move the agenda to new grounds.

RECONCEPTUALISING ADMINISTRATION, MANAGEMENT AND LEADERSHIP

Defining the nature of work carried out by early childhood professionals is not easy, even for those familiar with the field. Existing definitions have lacked clarity, coherence and comprehensiveness due to a failure to take into account changing circumstances and the consequent evolution of appropriate roles and responsibilities. Over time, writers have used a variety of terms to describe and discuss the roles and responsibilities of early childhood professionals (Clyde et al. 1994; Ebbeck 1991; Jalongo & Isenberg 2000; Smith & McMillan 1992). More recently, Oberhuemer (2000: 3) examined early childhood training programs in Europe, attempting to capture the emergent contours of a new role profile for those working with young children. Her list places a heavy emphasis on expanding the way early childhood professionals work with families, incorporating new dimensions such as father involvement, networking and quality assessment. It is interesting to compare these roles and responsibilities with those that were identified as 'common core elements' by the National Association for the Education of Young Children (NAEYC) in the USA (1993), as presented in Table 1.1.

It can be seen that both the NAEYC (1993) and Oberhuemer (2000) refer to management roles, but neither explicitly discusses leadership. The NAEYC's guidelines reflect conventional roles of early childhood professionals working

Table 1.1 Comparing common core elements with the emerging role profile of early childhood professionals

Common 'core' elements of early childhood professionals' work	Emerging profile of early childhood professionals in Europe
1. Demonstrate an understanding of child development and apply this knowledge in practice. 2. Observe and assess children's behaviour in planning and individualising teaching practices and curriculum. 3. Establish and maintain a safe and healthy environment for children. 4. Plan and implement a developmentally appropriate curriculum that advances all areas of children's learning and development. 5. Establish supportive relationships with children and implement developmentally appropriate techniques of guidance and group management. 6. Establish and maintain positive and productive relationships with families. 7. Support the development and learning of individual children, recognising that children are best understood in the context of family culture and society. 8. Demonstrate an understanding of the early childhood profession and make a commitment to professionalism.	1. Conceptualising and developing a program together with parents and local community input. 2. Presenting and legitimising professional practice with a lay audience. 3. Centre management, decision-making and administration of resources in a participatory manner. 4. Development of parent participation strategies for a wide range of families. 5. Development of specific strategies to facilitate father involvement, especially from minority ethnic families. 6. Networking: linking children's educational activities to broader community activities. 7. Supporting parent self-help groups. 8. Cooperating with other professionals regularly. 9. Examining and experimenting with diverse approaches to quality development and evaluation.

Sources: NAEYC (1993: 5), left column; Oberhuemer (2000), right column.

with children and families. Described as the 'core' elements, they reflect the fundamentals of early childhood practice that transcend various roles and settings in which professionals work. Taken together, 'the sum of the body of knowledge effectively distinguishes early childhood professionals from other professionals' (NAEYC 1993: 12). In contrast, dimensions of professional practice identified by Oberhuemer (2000: 3) extend these basics to include emergent responsibilities such as 'negotiating and networking competencies'.

Oberhuemer (2000: 3) is aware that early childhood professionals may view these functions as either a threat or an opportunity; accordingly, she concludes that:

> These emerging shifts in the practitioner's role are taking place in a context and climate of economic rationalism. The accompanying pressure of accountability is likely to produce an ambivalent stand among practitioners . . . The delicate interplay of contradictory forces needs to be recognised and addressed by both research and policy.

Table 1.2 Typology of an early childhood leader

Qualities	Skills	Roles and responsibiliites
• Kind, warm, friendly • Nurturant, sympathetic • Patient • Self-aware, rational, logical, analytical, knowledgeable • Goal-oriented, planful, assertive, proactive, professional, confident, visionary, influential	• Human resources management • Financial management • General administration • Effective communication • Technical competence as an early childhood professional in order to act as a model, guide and mentor	• To develop and articulate a philosophy, values and vision • To deliver a quality service • To engage in ongoing professional development and to encourage it in all staff • To be accountable and act as an advocate for children, parents, staff, the profession and the general community • To engage in a collaborative and partnership style of leadership • To be sensitive and responsive to the need for change and to manage change effectively

Source: Rodd (1996: 126).

Rodd (1996: 126) has attempted to identify the qualities, skills and leadership responsibilities of early childhood professionals, as shown in Table 1.2. Rodd's profile of an early childhood leader (1996) contains some similarities to Oberhuemer's (2000) conceptualisation of professional practice, as discussed. Rodd's typology of early childhood leaders is also more akin to the changing role of early childhood professionals working in modern Western societies such as Australia and the USA. However, this model also does not explicate the relationships between administration, management and leadership responsibilities in early childhood.

Table 1.3 represents our attempt to develop an integrated approach by exploring the relationships across the dispositions, skills and roles and responsibilities of administration, management and leadership in early childhood. With each ensuing chapter you are asked to see what elements can be framed against Table 1.3, as it provides a useful analysis to guide early childhood professionals working as administrators, managers or leaders.

The dispositions, skills and roles identified in Table 1.3 are not mutually exclusive to one sphere of activity such as administration, management or leadership. Instead, Table 1.3 is an attempt to provide a directional focus when undertaking various tasks, or when one or more of administration, management and leadership merge or become blurred into one role, position or job description. In some services, for instance, there may be one person who is responsible for all three roles. This person is commonly the centre director (sometimes referred to as the centre coordinator in Australia). It is not unusual for these individuals to experience a high level of stress in trying to respond to all demands simultaneously. It is thus not surprising that centre directors experience a high rate of early burnout (Goelman & Guo 1998; Rosier & Lloyd-Smith 1996; Sumsion 2002).

Organisational skills are the key to effective centre administration. It is often said that to be a good teacher you have to be organised. It is therefore usually assumed that all early childhood professionals have good organisational skills. The ability to organise and coordinate people, materials and space are all essential prerequisites in becoming a centre director. Yet research has shown clearly that, at the time of appointment as chief administrator of their centres, few, if any, have undertaken any formal training in the administrative (and management) responsibilities required of this position (Hayden 1996; Waniganayake et al. 1998).

Globalisation and changing political climates demand that we take charge of our destiny, and strong leadership is an effective tool for meeting the demands of these challenges. A review of the existing literature suggests that what we currently have is a highly structured approach to developing leadership in early childhood, one which is aligned to the position of centre directors. This means that leadership in early childhood is defined in terms of the position as a centre director and the functions or the roles and responsibilities required of these workers. This stance is not surprising given the links between the traditional orientation of leadership, administration and management. It is argued that such an approach is too restrictive, and does not take into account the diversity and complexity of the early childhood profession's demands in contemporary work environments. Our current understanding of leadership in early childhood is limited further because it does not encompass the sociocultural diversity and gender orientation of the field.

Table 1.3 Putting together administration, management and leadership

	Administration	Management	Leadership
Roles and responsibilities These are expected behaviours of a particular job or position, and may be specified in one's duty statement or job description.	• Maintain day-to-day tasks of data collection • Set up a system of records and files • Keep track of correspondence and financial dealings	• Monitor quality assessment and improvement • Analyse the needs of children, families and staff everyday • Oversee day-to-day financial upkeep.	• Facilitate staff development and training • Analyse the needs of children, families and staff from a long-term perspective • Design and direct policy development
Skills Learnt competencies acquired through training and experience, necessary to work as administrators, managers and leaders.	These are the technicalities or basic foundation competencies necessary for the organisation to function: • Awareness of official guidelines and legal requirements • Organisational skills such as documentation, correspondence and filing • Follows policies and procedures precisely	These are interactive skills necessary for maintaining a centre, and are concerned with immediate and short-term issues mainly: • Communication skills • Staff supervision and support • Marketing and promotion • Assessment and evaluation of programs, services and staff	Leadership skills relate to macro-level engagements, both inside and outside the centre, and are primarily concerned with the future: • Delegation • Research skills • Advocacy and lobbying • Liaison and networking • Policy formulation and analysis • Critical thinking
Dispositions Personal attributes or qualities of early childhood professionals that can affect their work. These may/may not vary according to each topic discussed in this book.	• Organised: approaches work systematically • Eager to obtain sound information • Demanding in searching for accuracy • Follows set policies and protocols • Comfortable with use of technology	• Understands the importance of accountability requirements • Enjoys working with staff and families • Concerned with risk assessment • Driven by efficiency and productivity • Entrepreneurial	• Enjoys working with others both within the centre and outside • Passionate about speaking out for children and families • Enjoys challenges • Visionary • Empowering • Articulatex • Adaptable

Of course, nothing remains static, and there is movement in the business world indicative of a need to reassess leadership theories that address contemporary challenges in that field. Much can be gained by looking at advances in theory and research across disciplines, as this provides new orientations or filtration systems against which to test our own views and beliefs about any aspect of knowledge and skills relevant to early childhood. To put it simply, to make someone who does not have an early childhood background, expertise or experience understand the professional's practices or theories, it is necessary to clarify and simplify the information needed, as ultimately this process will strengthen the professional's own goals and objectives. Accordingly, readers might consider the key leadership skills in Figure 1.6 as posed by Sarros and Butchatsky (1996: 284), which were based on a study of Australia's top chief executive officers in major corporations such as Telstra, Coca-Cola Amatil, McDonald's Australia and international banks.

Figure 1.6 Key leadership skills

Do you . . .

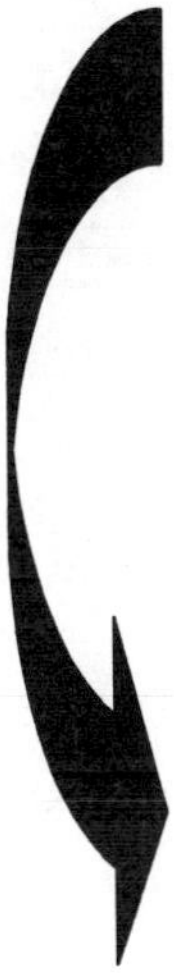

- have the ability to manage change?
- have a view of the future?
- seek out opportunities and challenge the status quo?
- involve everyone in developing organisational visions and mission statements?
- have the capacity to see the big picture?
- recruit the best people for the job?
- coach, mentor and role-model?
- understand the interaction between people and systems?
- ask questions and build on past achievements?
- align people to a cause?
- have knowledge of the business?
- manage time and responsibilities effectively?
- understand the need to balance conflicting constituencies?
- have mental toughness—conviction in your ability?

Do early childhood leaders need the same skills as those on this list or different skills?

Adapted from Sarros and Butchatsky (1996: 284).

Distributive leadership model

The question remains: what is the relationship between administration, management and leadership? In their book, when identifying the 'five faces of leadership', Kagan and Bowman (1997) partitioned administrative leadership from advocacy leadership and community leadership, and so on. The author responsible for writing the chapter on administrative leadership, Culkin, also separated management from leadership, but then went on to use administration and management interchangeably. Perhaps one of the more useful ways to explore this complexity is to consider the application of these three concepts—administration, management, leadership—within the children's centres that you know.

Waniganayake (2000) proposed a paradigm shift in reconceptualising leadership as a distributive phenomenon, and this model is illustrated in Figure 1.7.

Figure 1.7 DISTRIBUTIVE LEADERSHIP MODEL

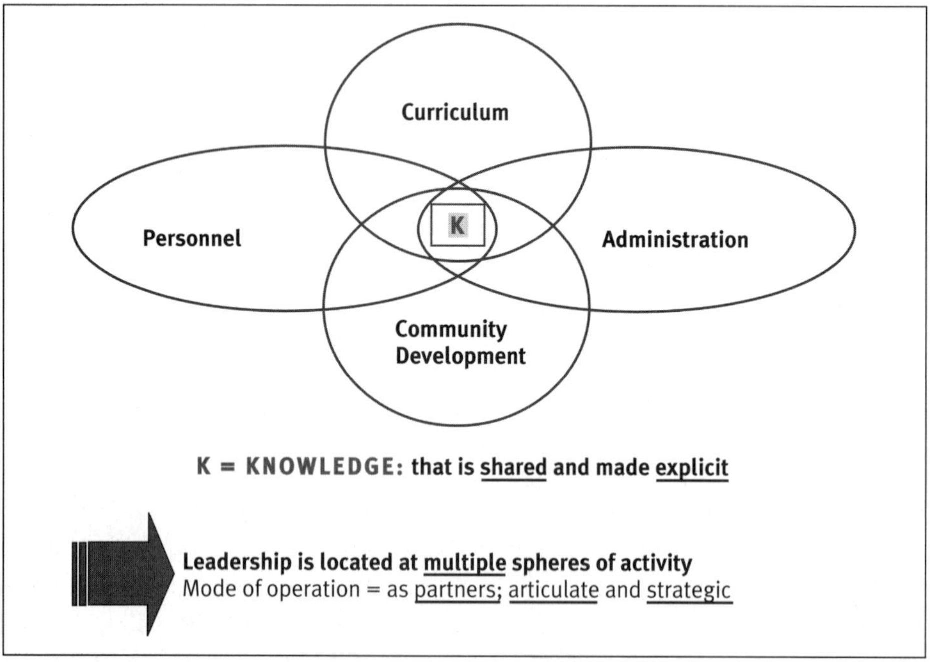

Source: Waniganayake (2000).

Within the distributive leadership model, knowledge is the central focus of organisational learning. Access to information and the ability to reflect, review and utilise this knowledge in appropriate ways, denote the early childhood professional's capacity to be a leader. Knowledge is therefore perceived as the foundation of leadership. Knowledge contains both pedagogical and practical understandings necessary to sustain and promote learning within the organisation from a long-term perspective. Leadership is acquired and nurtured by sharing knowledge in explicit ways. This is essential in articulating one's vision as a leader (Rodd, 1994, 1998). Knowledge may be specialised according to the functions, activities or services provided by the organisation such as whether it is a childcare centre or a family day care scheme, or a government department. Figure 1.7 depicts only one way that knowledge may be structurally dispersed within an organisation concerned with early childhood matters. In other words, this model can be adapted to accommodate differing specialisations that are possible within various early childhood settings.

By upholding diversity in leadership practice—be it in terms of style or strategies adopted by the leader, the distributive leadership model enables the realisation that there could be more than one leader within a single organisational setting. Figure 1.7, for instance, attempts to capture the existence of multiple leaders in a preschool or childcare setting. It shows that there could be four people working side by side with each specialising in terms of curriculum, personnel management, centre administration and outreach or community development work. These four specialists have leadership responsibilities for one particular area of expertise or domain of operation. For leadership to work in the organisational context, all four leaders need to come together in partnership, to articulate and build a cohesive and integrated plan of action that is meaningful and strategic to that organisation.

The distributive leadership model therefore draws us away from the single command and lead model characteristic of traditional leadership theory. It reflects a participatory and decentralised approach to leadership by locating leadership within multiple spheres of activity, where an individual with specific expertise and experience has the responsibility for guiding and coordinating activities with a particular focus. Given the increasing demands being placed on contemporary early childhood professionals working in rapidly changing societal contexts, it is argued that a specialist model such as the one depicted in Figure 1.7 would assist in gaining role clarity as well as a better sharing of complex responsibilities, particularly in centre based early childhood services.

In sum, the distributive leadership model relies on building relationships through recognition of existing knowledge and empowerment based on competence and understanding. It assumes that leadership cannot exist without knowledge or team work. Leadership is thus derived through creating a culture of learning and sustained by sharing knowledge in collaborative ways.

Future leadership challenges

Various authors have explored new pathways to leadership development, including links between training and leadership, roles of resource and referral agencies, mediating organisations as well as sharing leadership with parents (e.g. see Kagan & Bowman 1997; Sciarra & Dorsey 2002). This viewpoint is in keeping with Kagan and Bowman's thesis (1997) that leadership in early childhood is multifaceted and progress is based on inclusiveness of diverse interests, abilities and skills. Morgan (1997: 13) describes this as 'a set of reciprocal relationships'. There is a sense of sharing by early childhood leaders that departs from the single male focus of conventional leadership theories. It also encapsulates the importance of understanding the societal context of leadership that Sarros and Butchatsky (1996: 4) stated is necessary:

> *... taking the 'big picture' perspective of leadership helps balance the rhetoric with the reality, and serves to validate or refute the actions and attitudes of significant leaders.*

If one accepts the view of those such as Cox (1996) and Sinclair (1998) that leadership is inextricably gender-based, then given the fact that early childhood professionals are predominantly women, it is worthwhile considering the strategies for leadership achievement from a women's viewpoint. Cox (1996: 22) says that her objective is to redefine power and leadership from a woman's perspective so that women can own it and 'use power as a beneficial social change agent, without overlooking the potential of its darker side'.

By now it should be clear that leadership is socially constructed and involves the interaction with others and building of relationships over time. Yet there is one viewpoint that suggests that some people are born leaders. This view questions the nature–nurture arguments of leadership development (Waniganayake et al. 2000). Leadership research conducted over many decades does show that personal attributes and experience can influence the growth of leadership. Sarros and Butchatsky (1996), for example, found that background variables, including family characteristics, schooling and career experiences (e.g. role models and mentors), as well as personal attributes such as trust, vision, energy and decisiveness, were important in guiding leadership growth. For professionals interested in assessing their personal leadership style and attributes, there are many instruments and models available. One such example is the popular leadership assessment tool developed by Jorde-Bloom, Sheerer and Britz (1991b). Students may use this at the beginning of their training and retest themselves at the conclusion of training, to see whether there are any significant changes in the way they approach leadership matters.

Findings from the International Leadership Project (ILP) indicated that there is an urgent need to review the ways in which professionals conceptualise leadership in early childhood (Waniganayake et al. 2000). A comparison of findings from Finland and Australia helps to illustrate the cross-cultural nature of leadership challenges in diverse societies (see Table 1.4). In both countries, early childhood professionals faced challenges involving philosophical, pedagogical and political concerns. The methods used in tackling these challenges were, however, not fully explored in this study. By comparing and contrasting these findings with Sarros and Butchatsky's list of future challenges (1996: 284–5) as identified in Figure 1.8, the extent to which there is compatibility across disciplines can be assessed.

These leadership challenges (Figure 1.8), when viewed in association with

Table 1.4 Major issues confronting early childhood professionals in Australia and Finland

In Australia . . .	In Finland . . .
• Low professional status and poor public image • Sectional interests—lack of unity within the profession • Pedagogical concerns over program quality • Training reform—debates over core knowledge • Philosophical concerns—place of children and women in society • Government reforms and impact of funding cuts • Linking research and policy reform	• Low professional status • Decision-making about limited resources • Concerns about daycare centre staff wellbeing • Establishing connections between policy, politics and practice • Reconciliation of comprehensive and integrated leadership with disconnected power and responsibility

Source: Waniganayake and Hujala (2001).

Figure 1.8 Future leadership challenges

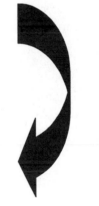

- Competing more successfully on the global stage
- Keeping pace with technology
- Satisfying client needs
- Systematic leadership throughout the organisation
- Maintaining an excellent staff
- Increased returns to shareholders
- Emphasis on core company values
- Creating a team-based culture
- Maintaining patience
- Succession planning
- Refocusing direction and strategic planning
- Environmental responsibility

How do these challenges affect early childhood organisations?

Adapted from Sarros and Butchatsky (1996: 284–5).

the profile statements developed by the NAEYC (1993) and Oberhuemer (2000) and discussed earlier, show very clearly the importance of embracing a wider world view in exploring the professionals' roles and responsibilities as leaders in early childhood. Sarros and Butchatsky's list brings together the basics of customer satisfaction and team spirit, with the broader concerns of the environment and the global marketplace. Even for the early childhood professionals there is no escape from globalisation, and we discuss this in detail in Chapter 8. Technology can be harnessed effectively in designing and creating a strategic plan of action to implement leadership visions. If the early childhood professional's goal is to create sustainable communities we need leadership to make it happen, and early childhood professionals are well placed to take on this role.

Participation in leadership discussions as early childhood professionals is critical to advancing one's own professional development as well as the future development of the profession as a whole. As Sarros and Butchatsky (1996: 3) contend:

> Children are the best reminders that leadership takes more than just talent and innate skills. Leadership also takes a heck of a lot of patience, commitment to a cause, and the ability to acknowledge the views of others even when those views may be contrary to your own. So from this perspective, leadership rests firmly in the promotion of others' abilities and strengths while maintaining a dispassionate acceptance of the fact that by encouraging this growth in others, you are making yourself redundant.

CHAPTER SUMMARY

This chapter has attempted to deal with the complex concepts of administration, management and leadership as related to early childhood contexts:

- The low status and poor image of early childhood professionals has been discussed with reference to current research.
- Organisational contexts have been discussed in relation to administration, management and leadership.
- Leadership has been defined and typologies presented with relevance to early childhood contexts.
- New directions and obstacles to leadership have been outlined.
- A framework for reconceptualising administration, management and leadership has been presented and readers are challenged to apply this to the ensuing chapters.

   Discussion and reflection

1. Write and collate a series of definitions used to describe administration, management and leadership. Analyse these definitions in terms of the differences and similarities between the three concepts. Do the definitions

accurately convey the author's meaning? Explore why it may/may not be necessary or important to distinguish between these three concepts.

2. Draw the organisational structure of the centre best known to you. Clearly define who was reporting to whom, and for what purpose.

    (a)   What are the strengths and weaknesses of this organisational chart?
    (b)   Does the division of roles and responsibilities in this centre facilitate or hinder the centre's overall administration and management?

3. In one short sentence, how would you describe to someone who does not know anything about the early childhood field what you do as an early childhood professional? What key words or phrases would you use?

4. Do you agree with the model of distributive leadership presented in this book? Give reasons. If you agree that leadership in early childhood is a multifaceted phenomenon, are there other dimensions of leadership that we should consider? Describe these.

5. Reflecting on your own skills, knowledge and personal preferences, consider the challenges of implementing the distributive leadership model in your place of employment.

Chapter 2

Responding to change through effective management and leadership

This chapter is concerned primarily with change and the change process in organisations. It also considers how management confronts change, manages change or, indeed, leads change. Every organisation, whether public or private, profit-making or non profit-making, requires some form of management, and it is usually seen that the success of an organisation correlates with the quality of its managers. Change is looked at here from theoretical perspectives and then specifically in the applied context of early childhood.

Outcomes

At the conclusion of this chapter, the reader should have:

- developed an understanding of some theoretical perspectives on change;
- some understanding of the process of change;
- related the process of change to early childhood contexts;
- developed an understanding of the role of the early childhood leader in managing change;
- some knowledge of how to apply change to everyday early childhood contexts.

The following is a typical example of a change confronting an early childhood professional in Singapore. What are some of the theories behind change that can help when confronting a change like the one documented in Case study 2.1?

Case study 2.1
Change introduced by management

The director of a large early childhood centre in Singapore sought to effect some change to the way staff reported to management and parents on the children's progress. She set out to move the staff away from a teacher-directed, prescribed curriculum driven by preconceptions of parental and societal pressure for academic excellence to one that was child-centred. The director believed that the current use or misuse by staff of observation techniques only exacerbated the problems inherent in a centralised curriculum that was academically oriented. Observations were not used as the basis of program planning in the centre's programs and reporting to parents followed a set, somewhat rigid practice based on assessed achievement of set tasks.

The process of change involved 15 teachers in the centre over a period of eight weeks. It was, in many ways, a process of staff development, as staff were involved fully both in the data gathering on which decisions could be made for proposed changes and in self-analysis of the outcomes. The outcomes described below showed that, when given the opportunity in a climate of support, teachers could change their belief system through the construction of their own knowledge. Teachers began to question their preconceptions of the children, their practice and the school's adherence to its comprehensive, academic report in the form of a checklist.

Of course, what this study shows is that, in instances such as the one described, the changing of the teachers' perceptions and practices was only the beginning of the change needed. Some sort of balance and reconciliation between the teachers' views and those of the parents participating in the system also had to be worked on.

Observations and evaluations made by the teachers on the effectiveness of the change process were interesting. As the use of the then current checklist style of reporting to parents was one of the key issues governing the teachers' observation practices their comments, on reflection, indicated that while the practice was *more or less adequate* for parents it was *less than adequate* for teachers. It was considered more useful if used as a benchmark, as all areas of the curriculum were covered. The main disadvantage as reported was, in the teachers' own words: 'I don't think they (school reports) are looked at once they're done', 'It's just a tick box and we just do it, not really with the intention of monitoring the child', 'It does not tell how well a child can do' and so on.

Evaluating the change process in relation to training in the use of observations, the majority of staff felt confident in using this strategy as a basis for curriculum development. All teachers felt that its use would have a positive effect on their knowledge and understanding of the children. Concern remained as to how to

Continued

extract knowledge from these observations, and it was accepted that this should be the subject of ongoing staff development.

As the objective of the change process was to get teachers to see their observation techniques and reporting practices in a new light, it could be claimed that the change was achieved. However, as with all changes of this magnitude (as it was levelled at the core of teaching beliefs and practice), the process described here was but the first step in a much deeper and more significant change. Teachers in the process claimed that as a result of changing their observation practices they saw the children in a different light. One teacher commented:

> *I have a better understanding of the whole child now. In the past, before I used this technique [observations], I just tested them on specific areas and all I knew was that particular area [curriculum] at that point in time. When you are doing an observation, you observe the same child over a longer period of time and can make adjustments to what you observe and I think your understanding just gets better over time.*

The initial findings in relation to how the parents saw the *changed* parent–teacher conferences were surprising, in that the majority of parents saw very little difference. Most parents were content to know that their child was *right there in the middle for the year group, right there with the rest of the kids, not below.* What might be difficult for the staff in subsequent interviews, when they change their method of reporting (as a consequence of the newly adopted observational techniques) to that of a 'portfolio method', will be a subject for further staff development.

Used with the permission of Zee Kavanagh 2001, Singapore.

Case study 2.1 is one of change initiated by management in an early childhood centre. It shows how the process of introducing a change can be successful if done cooperatively, as free of threat as possible and with optimum support. It also highlights the necessity in large-scale, system-wide change for ongoing support, direction and related staff development.

Some theoretical issues relating to change

Managers do more than merely 'turn on switches' to make things work and work well. Management is a very complex task, even for small organisations such as a childcare centre with several staff and a (relatively) small number of children (clients) like that mentioned in Case study 2.1. In education, the individual school is an organisation and, for management purposes, must be seen as one. School systems also are organisations, which behave differently from their components (the individual schools) because they have different roles and responsibilities.

Throughout this chapter:

- Change is an ever-present entity: in fact, it is a necessity in all dynamic organisations. Here 'dynamic' implies continued growth to meet existing and future demand.
- An organisation can choose to change or not change. Its decision will be reflected in its survival. During periods of growth, organisations can be seen to be evolutionary, progressive and striving to change. Sometimes this change is revolutionary, especially when revolutionary methods are necessary for survival.
- Many childcare centres throughout Australia and elsewhere have gone through what they would describe as revolutionary changes as they have fought for their survival in a changing environment. In most cases the changes thrust on the early childhood sector have not been accompanied by essential—certainly desirable—support systems to prepare the workers for the changes.
- Many, if not most, schools and school systems have undergone what might be seen as radical changes to their curricula. In early childhood services there have been major changes as elements of preschool services have been joined to school services with subsequent management redirections. In child care, the input of preschooling and before- and after-school-hours care for older children has caused a change in the way that care centres operate. These are but a few examples of change that have influenced educational services in recent times.
- Change is all about us all, whether we like it or not. If we accept that change is necessary to our survival, if we react to it, adapt to it and manage it within current cultural, political and economic systems, then what we do in our early childhood establishments and how we do it may guarantee our continued survival, for a time at least. Management has to be ready for change as well as be ready to change.

The management of change is embedded in organisational theory. Both theory and management have changed over time. Hodge and Johnson (1988, in Razik & Swanson 2001: 41) described a taxonomy of six analytical models of management: mechanistic/bureaucratic, human relations, individual behaviour, technological, economic, and power. Razik and Swanson (2001: 41) go on to say that these models proceed from several assumptions:

- The organisation exists to satisfy environmental needs.
- The organisation's work system mobilises to meet objectives that will in turn meet environmental needs.
- The organisation structures itself to facilitate the work system activity.

- The design of power and authority relationships, system differentiation, and delegation are all dedicated to work facilitation.
- Renewal and change processes are mandatory for survival and effectiveness.

From the early models of management we can describe open and dynamic management as being interrelated across functional boundaries and integrating the various combinations of interactive processes. The necessity for interdependence between systems and subsystems in an organisation is critical in management, otherwise the organisation begins to resemble a conglomerate in which the reasonably autonomous systems and subsystems (components) are independent of each other. What we are considering here are organisations that are not mega-sized conglomerates but are rather those whose internal structures interrelate and interact. People in such organisations are the key element in achieving these processes. Management must therefore be concerned about the people in the process, particularly their perceptions of change.

Using the ideas of Kimborough and Nunnery (1998), Razik and Swanson (2001: 40) write that in a thriving organisation or system:

> ... individuals ... move from immaturity towards maturity, from passive to active, dependent to independent, now-oriented to future-oriented, from external to internal locus of control, and from a limited to a profound sense of commitment.

The above statement reflects those goals that all good management practices should aim for, as building up the strengths and commitment of the people in an organisation can only result in organisational growth. Thriving organisations have a realistic balance between the elements of bureaucracy and innovation, where bureaucracy refers to those elements of management necessary to keep the daily functioning of the organisation operating (e.g. routines, rules, regulations). Innovation, on the other hand, refers to how the organisation responds in a flexible, adaptable way to external demands (e.g. new accreditation requirements, staffing ratio changes).

The word 'systems' has been introduced several times so far in this brief discussion on management. What does the term 'systems' mean? Embedded in organisational theory is the systems approach to analysing management models in the social arena, of which education is part. One of the advantages to considering systems theory is that as the boundaries of systems are continually redefined by events in the systems or their environment, management practices can shift successfully to meet these changing boundaries.

SYSTEMS THEORY

- Back as far as 1938, Barnard viewed an organisation as 'a system of consciously co-ordinated activities of two or more persons' (1938: 73). This early definition includes key words that help in understanding what an organisational system is.
- According to Steers and Black, implications are there that the organisation has stated goals and purposes, a communication system, other coordinating processes and a network of individuals who cooperate on tasks for achieving the organisation's purposes (1994: 322).

What we see in these definitions and others (see also the dictionary for a definition of 'system') is that organisations are made up of groups of people working together to achieve common goals. This idea and its accompanying concept are quite different from seeing a system as an aggregate of units. What is missing here is the interactivity, mentioned earlier, of each of the aggregates and the integrating agent that brings them together.

Discussion on systems theory usually distinguishes between closed systems, where everything is produced and consumed solely within the system, and open systems, where inputs are received from an external environment and outputs are returned to the external environment. Seeing systems in such a way, as either closed or open, is more theoretical than practical. Razik and Swanson (2001: 32) indicate that theorists speak of relative closure or openness. Relatively closed systems need new energy as input so as to overcome entropy. The term 'relatively open systems' refers to degrees of openness. Such systems are exposed to many interventions, interruptions, interferences—some deliberatively sought, others not foreseen. The relatively closed systems may be psychologically comforting, as unwarranted intrusions are guarded against and any threat of change is derailed. The relatively open systems are exposed to external interventions, they can reach beyond their stated boundaries to exact external influence, there may be a degree of excitement created by dynamic movement, and other kinds of benefits may be enjoyed. Self-regulatory devices may be established to monitor any proposed changes to the system (Razik & Swanson 2001: 32). The characteristics of a more open system are interrelationship, interaction and interdependence (2001: 33).

The systems theory model favoured by Razik and Swanson (2001: 38) adds another dimension to the classical Input–Throughput–Output or the Input–Throughput–Output–Feedback models. Feedback is seen to contribute to the self-regulatory process that detects needed change. Razik and Swanson see the importance of the environment as a factor in influencing both the throughput and output stages. Here, the environment refers to 'the collection

Figure 2.1 Permeable system boundary

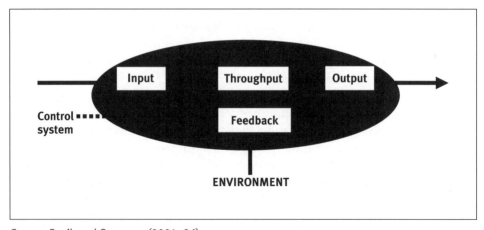

Source: Razik and Swanson (2001: 36).

of systems that lie outside the system under study . . . [which] are not con-trollable by the system but can be selectively responsive to the system's behav-iour' (2001: 37). Their model is diagrammed in Figure 2.1.

For systems growth to occur there must be quality human, technological and organisational inputs from within and outside the system. The factors of energy, interactivity and interdependence mentioned before must be there as well. This model represents the milieu in which most schools and early child-hood organisations operate, and it is the systems theory that underlies much of the analysis of the effectiveness of these organisations.

There has been some discussion in educational circles during the past decade as to planning for change using a futures scenario (Beare & Slaughter 1994; Toffler 1990). As Razik and Swanson (2001: 46) state:

> *Scenario planning and plotting is a new strategic process that holds the potential to revise how educational practitioners create change. Being able to deal with problems associated with some future scenario is wholly different from dealing with existing circumstances from a current or historical frame of reference(s).*

If we accept that education leads change—and we should, if we believe that the more educated we become the more concerned we are that certain change is desirable—then we should be futures-oriented in our thinking, planning and educating. This is what the change process is all about.

CHANGE AS A PROCESS

Over the past 20 years there has been considerable unrest and change in Australia's early childhood services, some of it being stimulated by the early childhood professionals themselves wanting to do things better, but much of it coming from political pressure for 'accountability', in both cost and quality. Here, the politicians justify their desires for change in terms of getting the maximum value for the taxpayer's dollar. In another context, they see it as an attempt to overcome what communities and nations believe are falling standards of care and education.

The reasons for change in education are complex and the ramifications of such change are far-reaching. Prerequisites to change are familiarity with the environment, willingness and ability to change, and acceptance of information and feedback (Schoderbek, Schoderbek & Kefalas 1990). It is essential that early childhood teachers, in particular, understand the process of change, for they are the ones at the forefront of change and implementing these changes in their daily workplace.

Rodd (1998: 127) says, of change in early childhood, that it:

- is inevitable;
- is necessary;
- is a process;
- occurs in individuals, organisations and societies;
- can be anticipated and planned for;
- is a highly emotional process;
- can cause tension and stress;
- is resisted by many people;
- can be adjusted to by individuals and groups with the support of the leader;
- entails developmental growth in attitudes and skills, policies and procedures; and
- is best facilitated on the basis of diagnosed needs.

It was Toffler (1990) who said that the 'survival of the fastest' will be the hallmark of the 21st century. The 'fastest' are those with the ability to shorten development times, to move products and services faster and closer to consumers, and to use information almost instantaneously (Razik & Swanson 2001: 44).

THE CHANGING EARLY CHILDHOOD WORKPLACE

Early childhood services have become increasingly diverse, and the changes to management structures, staffing requirements, client needs—to name but a few elements in early childhood services—have challenged leaders to respond positively and in some instances quickly if their particular service is to survive financially and educationally.

The cost factor

The competitive aspect of providing services is a relatively new (since the 1970s) phenomenon and one which some services, both private (commercial) and community-based, have not been able to respond to effectively. Competition comes mainly from two causes: cost of the service, and quality of the service.

The demand for child care, for example, is likely to remain, even grow modestly; however, the client group is now much more discerning than it was 20 years ago when there were not enough services and places to match the demand. The increase in the number of private and community providers, again in both preschools and childcare services, has exacerbated this competitive element, as not all expansion of services has been planned. The result of such poor planning, if any, has been that in some localities (mainly in urban areas) there is an oversupply of provision, and centres have to resort to a variety of strategies to attract clients. While there are always problems when competitive elements are introduced into a service provision, there are also positive and healthy outcomes. There is nothing wrong with good competition, as it keeps the services operating within realistic bounds with some consideration given to quality.

Many professionals do not like to see the term 'industry' applied to early childhood services. However, one does have to look beyond government models of social services to areas of industry to find examples of high-quality, efficient and financially viable services, irrespective of the specific label on the work being done, or the service provider. One thing is certain: the days of being insulated from change have gone, probably never to return.

QUALITY ISSUES

Another driving force that has brought about positive change in early childhood services has been the identification of, need and concern for better quality in service provision. The concern for quality in early childhood services is worldwide. It is not simply a byproduct of the resources available but, as Woodhead (1996: 92) says:

> ... reflects the widely differing social contexts into which early childhood programmes are embedded ... (the child-rearing beliefs and practices of parents and

the broader community, family networks, schools) which shape what is valuable
for early childhood and how it can be achieved.

The desire to improve quality is very much central to the social thrusts of most countries—developed as well as less developed. Quality is, however, a relative concept, and its dimensions vary greatly according to the cultural context.

In Hong Kong, for example, the government has put more resources into the training of early childhood staff so that the quality of teaching in early childhood centres will be improved. Minimum standards of training, including length and level of courses, have been changed. From 1995 there have been bachelor's-degree-level courses in early childhood development in Hong Kong. In Singapore, in 2001, early childhood diplomas were mandated by government ministries as a required level of training for staff in charge of early childhood centres. Degree-level courses are not considered necessary at this time for early childhood teaching in Singapore. Such developments in the training of early childhood staff will, one hopes, influence positively the quality of programs offered in early childhood centres, and further government-led developments in training/educating will have spin-off effects on quality.

Improvements in the quality of service provision in long-day care in Australia have been noted since the implementation in 1993 of the National Childcare Accreditation Council's (NCAC) Quality Improvement and Accreditation System (QIAS). While the accreditation system initially was directed towards centre-based long-day care, it was widened in 2001 to include family day care—a style of care provided by adults (usually mothers) in their homes for up to six children (depending on licensing requirements). (Readers interested in the QIAS and the Australian National Childcare Accreditation Council's work can gain detailed information from the NCAC's website at http://www.ncac.gov.au.)

It is appropriate here to note that the QIAS is based on the process of self-study, which is counterchecked by an external colleague (peer) working in child care. Quality is based on a number of 'principles' (35 in number) that serve as indicators of quality and are grouped under 10 'quality areas'. This basis underwent a revision during 1999 and 2000, as it was felt that the initial system had served its purpose well but after some seven years of operation was ready for a review and revision. The second edition of the QIAS handbook (NCAC 2001b: 4) notes:

> *Quality improvement is a collaborative process involving those who have the most interest in the quality of care. The QIAS encourages each centre and its families to work together in their complementary roles to define a philosophy and goals to guide the program, the style of interactions and all other activities at the centre.*

We believe that the process of self-study and the collaborative nature of it are the strengths of this quality improvement and accreditation system. It is not an 'inspectorial' system, such as can be found in many school systems and which evaluates standards for individual centres/schools. Rather, in analysing and evaluating its own efforts each centre grows in knowledge and understanding of what quality is all about and is able to put the quality indicators into local and cultural perspectives (Ebbeck 2001: 5).

THE WORKFORCE AND CHANGE

The issues of employee motivation and commitment are related to level of training, status, and other industrial issues such as remuneration, holiday entitlements and other employee entitlements.

It is well known that the status of early childhood professionals and para-professionals throughout the world is lower than for most other sectors in what might be referred to as 'the human services'. The status of childcare 'workers' *vis-à-vis* preschool teachers is markedly different. The lower status of the childcare worker brings with it a considerably lower salary, longer working hours, shorter holidays and often greatly reduced tenure.

The 'tenure' aspect, or lack of it, in child care (at least in Australia) is one of the greatest contributors to low morale in the workforce and less than optimal commitment to the job. In saying this, it should be noted that childcare staff, in general, are committed to their work and to the welfare of the children in their care. However, the less than optimal conditions mentioned here as compared with their counterparts in other services cannot help but affect the morale and commitment of many in the workforce.

Allied to staff motivation and commitment is a high turnover of staff, particularly among the more junior and untrained staff in child care, coupled with a high level of stress and burnout.

One cannot deny that employees represent any organisation's single biggest asset. This statement is particularly relevant to the human services sector. Most kindergartens (if they are not part of a larger school complex) are small enterprises, with staff often numbering fewer than six persons. Childcare centres also are small enterprises, though the staffing numbers might be slightly larger because of the extended hours of operation and licensing requirements for the ratio of staff to children. If staff morale here is low and staff's commitment to their work questionable the result is in the main an unhappy centre, with a high turnover of staff and poor-quality services. Of course, the poor quality often means centres going out of business as their clients go to where quality is obvious.

Rodd (1998: 132) used Dunphy's (1986) description of individuals in organisations as being along a continuum: on one end were 'learning persons', and on the other 'self-defeating persons'. The learning person sees change as an opportunity for growth and development, whereas the self-defeating person believes that change threatens his/her sense of security and may demand skills that he/she does not possess.

- A person's self-esteem is most influential to his/her productivity, however this may be manifested.
- A person with a low self-esteem who is not supported in a positive way so as eventually to build up his/her self-esteem cannot, in times of change, be a fully functioning person.
- Self-esteem, in this sense, has to do with capacity—to accept change, to accommodate it—to function as a productive member of a staff team. It does not refer to a person's cautiousness in questioning purposes of and methods used in change processes. These behaviours can be seen in a positive light, as being strategies for clarifying purposes and processes, even to the point of introducing possible alternatives.

NEW TECHNOLOGIES AND CHANGE

Early childhood services are now beginning to use technologies in the workplace, not only in management activities but also in the curriculum planned and implemented for children. When one considers the spectrum of education from secondary to early childhood teaching, the last to become proficient with the new available technologies has probably been early childhood.

It is hoped that the increased use of technologies will make early childhood administration and teaching more efficient and dynamic and that advances will continue to be made. It is essential that teachers are willing to respond to the exciting and positive changes that appropriate technology can bring to early childhood for, if used wisely, these can only improve the quality of service provision.

DIVERSITY OF AND IN SERVICES—ANOTHER CHANGE

Since the mid-1970s in Australia early childhood services, namely childcare and kindergarten/preschool, have changed considerably. Prior to that time child care was largely the responsibility of the private sector, where care centres operated on a profit-making basis. Fees were paid by families to the centre operators for the care given. It was very much a commercial enterprise. Kindergartens/preschools also were operated largely outside the formal school systems, but most were community-based and non-profit enterprises.

During the 1970s considerable government funding was allocated to early childhood services, both child care and preschooling, as a consequence of new government policies and priorities that were both politically and economically driven. Government-funded child care came into existence in competition with the private sector; the training of childcare personnel was formalised within the technical and further education colleges; and, as a result, new regulations and standards of care were established. Preschooling was practically wholly government-funded, in keeping with election promises of free preschool education for every child for the year prior to entering formal schooling. This action also saw the beginning of preschools attached to primary schools and the assumption of responsibility for preschooling by education ministries and education departments.

The above activity has led to a total revamping of early childhood services in less than 30 years. While this may sound like a long time, in reality it is not long when one considers the enormity of the change experienced. The people working in the early childhood field would say that change brings further change. There are always things to be done differently—management and curriculum. Government intervention, funding and policy making all bring new demands, new requirements for management and accountability. (Some of these issues are picked up later in this chapter.)

WHY CHANGE?

So far in this chapter the discussion has related directly to those factors central to change in the early childhood workplace. These factors are no different from those in general industry, as all industry is made up of people and their practices. Sometimes people think of industry first as machinery and technology and only second as people, yet it is the people who make up any organisation. When change is in the air it is the people who become tense, who have fears (or generate them) of the unknown, who have their security of both mind and body threatened. This section deals with the people in the process of change and their behaviour during the change process.

The basic answer to the question 'Why change?' is that if we did not change we would be left behind, as the change that is going on around us will continue whether we participate in it and embrace it or not. It has always been believed that education causes change: the more educated a person or society, the more possibilities will become evident. 'Possibilities' here means 'potential'. Such a belief is based on the idea that education is a forward-looking enterprise, that it directs change, it leads the process of change. If only this were true. More often than not now change (particularly societal and technological change) is leading educational practices, and it is a matter of education catching up.

Fullan (1982) wrote that change can either aggravate the teacher's problem or provide a glimmer of hope.

Change can, therefore, be both positive and negative:

- How teachers cope with change is extremely important.
- Often change is something hurried.
- If it is not fully understood by those people responsible for its implementation (the staff), its implementation can be more damaging than productive.

In 1961 Chin, Bennis and Benne wrote their now classic book, *The Planning of Change*. A number of subsequent revisions have not changed the authors' central thesis on change:

> *Living in an age whose single constant is change, all men and women are in urgent need of whatever resources can be made available as they seek to understand and manage themselves and their environments, to understand and solve the unprecedented personal and social problems that confront them.*
>
> *The intellectual challenge comes from the necessity to develop an adequate theory of the processes through which knowledge of human behaviour and of human systems is applied and utilised. More particularly, a theory of applying and adapting theories of social, interpersonal, and personal dynamics to the special case of deliberate changing is required.   (Bennis, Benne & Chin 1985: 111)*

They go on to say that part of the practical challenge of implementing change is to help people develop as effective and responsible agents of planned change. One can approve or deplore change but no-one can deny its importance, and we all need to have a greater understanding of the potential and limitations of any change:

> *Richard Weaver once remarked that the ultimate term in contemporary rhetoric, the 'god term', is 'process' or 'change': the world, as Oppenheimer remarks, alters as we walk in it. It would appear, then, that we are beyond debating the inevitability of change; most students of our society agree that the one major invariant is the tendency toward movement, growth, development, process: change. The contemporary debate has swung from change versus no change to methods employed in controlling and directing forces in change. Dewey has remarked that '. . . history in being a process of change generates change not only in details but also in the method of directing social change'.   (Bennis, Benne & Chin 1985: 2)*

Teachers, parents and adults generally say that today's children know more about more things, have experienced many more things and have internalised these experiences within a very different 'mindset' from that of previous generations. If our curricula in schools and early childhood settings were not to change, we would be doing our children a considerable disservice.

Figure 2.2 The change continuum

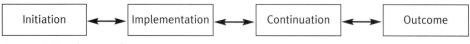

Source: Fullan (1991: 48).

All these positives for change notwithstanding, change simply for the sake of change is illogical. We see such change from time to time as a result of political whims and fancies, especially after political elections. It is an offshoot of the 'new broom sweeping clean' mentality. Pressure groups within organisations come and go but while they have influence and a power of sorts they can propose change, instigate it and often lead it. A good example in early education at present is the rise in the influence of curricula based on the 'constructivist' approach. Influential pressure groups within educational authorities that support what they see as curricular reform instigate great change in schooling and early childhood systems. However, what is not generally appreciated is that many approaches—the constructivist approach in this case— have been around for a long time. The constructivist approach, together with the 'project method', formed the basis for John Dewey's work during the early 1900s in the USA. Such approaches are helpful, and lead to positive change when they are seen as guidelines or proposals. When they become prescriptions to be followed they lose their effectiveness and individuality for curriculum, and teaching methods are based on a very personal belief system and concept of professionalism.

Fullan (1991) wrote that change is a process, not an isolated single event, and it occurs over time. The simplified graph of the change process is shown in Figure 2.2. In explaining this continuum, Fullan (1991) proposes that either someone or a group initiates a need for change:

- The implementation process then begins and the continuation phase is an extension beyond the initial period.
- The outcome phase refers to different types of results, and these will vary greatly.
- It is important to note the two-way arrows in the diagram, as it is not a straight, linear process, and events can alter decisions taken at any phase.
- The time perspective will vary greatly depending on the scope of the change.
- Whatever happens at one phase is likely to influence and affect subsequent stages, and new determinants are likely to appear.

CHANGE WITHIN ORGANISATIONS

Most literature on change divides any analysis of the change process into factors that are external and those that are internal to the organisation experiencing the change, no matter how large or small that organisation. For example, in early childhood services in Australia the recent removal of the government administration subsidy previously allocated to community-based childcare centres required a great deal of rethinking by centre administration and management of its administrative practices, staffing profile, its fee structure—in fact the centre's total program. This example illustrates that in small operations (and childcare centres are small operations when compared with the world of business generally) the removal of a relatively small sum (such as $A40000 p.a.) can generate quite a considerable degree of change within that operation.

A further example of organisational change in early childhood services could be the consolidation within one administrative structure of what was previously a separate, community-based kindergarten and an adjoining or nearby primary school. In such cases—and there have been quite a number of kindergartens integrated into primary school complexes in Australia—there would be first the necessity for acceptance by the new administrative authority of the two different yet complementary activities under its jurisdiction. There would be a non-compulsory element (kindergarten) and a compulsory element (schooling), with differing funding models or criteria (yet with realistic equity in treatment). Second, and continually, there would be considerations of a curricular nature (e.g. the continuity between kindergarten for 3–5-year-olds and that of primary schooling for the over-5s). There would be differences in the philosophical underpinnings of the nature and curricula of the two services, probably differences in styles and methods of reporting to parents and so on. The early childhood personnel who have gone through such structural changes in the past would agree that the process, while perhaps desirable in the long run, has not necessarily been easy or smooth in the initial stages.

The two examples of change in early childhood presented here are examples of change stemming from external factors. In the first example the factor was government policy changes (financing). In the second example, again the factor was government intervention but probably with a degree of local, community consultation. In early childhood services generally, as with most of the human services, change is often stimulated by a result of government action, of either a policy or a funding nature.

While some of the changes listed above are seen to be stimulated by 'internal factors', there is often also an external element behind the change. However, the underlying criterion in such cases is that it is the forces within the organisation (staff, management, parents) that make the decision to change, that structure the change process and support it.

Often the change stimulated from within an organisation is reflected in the changing of routines to meet changing demands. Such change can be as minor as altering a daily time schedule to accommodate a one-off activity, such as a visiting entertainment group. Or it can be a relatively major change, as when dividing large groups of children into smaller units according to age so that staff allocation can better suit the experience and expertise of the staff.

Differentiation has to be made between routine change and change brought about unexpectedly by a crisis, such as the illness and non-attendance of staff. Early childhood establishments face this kind of change every day and have usually developed contingency measures, such as a relief staff procedure, to meet their immediate needs.

From the aforementioned discussion and examples of change in early childhood organisations it should be clear that change is one of the few certainties in daily life and management. The process of change can be smooth or troublesome. It can be accepted by staff positively, or it can be resisted. Either way it creates stress, which must be dealt with by staff and particularly by the leader.

RESISTANCE TO CHANGE

Again, most of the literature on managing change discusses resistance to change from two perspectives: that of resistance stemming from personal sources (i.e. from the perspective of the personnel within an organisation), and that of organisational resistance. Table 2.1 lists the personal and organisational reasons for resistance to change. It is taken from a text on organisational behaviour and shows numerous reasons for resistance.

Personal—or, indeed, personnel—resistance comes about as the result of a number of the factors listed in Table 2.1. While there may be a number of reasons why resistance to change is a factor in early childhood services, with sound leadership over time such resistance is generally overcome. If there is too much change, the changes being introduced too often or in such large steps that they become 'indigestible' and difficult to manage, resistance may be prolonged. Where there is a degree of passive resistance among staff the process of change will be slowed down. Where this happens in organisations the task of the leader in the change process becomes more complicated. In the main, personal resistance comes about as a result of fearing the unknown and this, in personnel management terms, is quite understandable. Fear also brings with it a degree of stress, and with stress comes pressure placed on staff.

Stressful situations do not make for harmony within an organisation, and when the workplace is seen by staff to be counter to their ideal (of what it

Table 2.1 Personal and organisational reasons for change

Personal sources	Organisational sources
1. Misunderstanding of purpose, mechanics, or consequences of change 2. Failure to see need for change 3. Fear of unknown 4. Fear of loss of status, security, power etc. resulting from change 5. Lack of identification or involvement with change 6. Habit 7. Vested interests in status quo 8. Group norms and role prescriptions 9. Threat to existing social relationships 10. Conflicting personal and organisational objectives	1. Reward system may reinforce status quo 2. Interdepartmental rivalry or conflict, leading to an unwillingness to cooperate 3. Sunk costs in past decisions and actions 4. Fear that change will upset current balance of power 5. Prevailing organisational climate 6. Poor choice of method of introducing change 7. Past history of unsuccessful change attempts and their consequences 8. Structural rigidity

Source: Steers and Black (1994: 669).

could and should be), then the staff look for something to blame or for an excuse for their actions. If change is in the making, it becomes a target for the staff's hostility.

The leader in any change situation has to be wary, as passive resistance can easily go 'underground'. Whatever the symptoms and apparent causes of the resistance might be, these must be kept out in the open so that they can be dealt with openly by all involved.

Organisational resistance in early childhood services is difficult to sustain, as the continued existence of such services is dependent on funding—which, in Australia, comes largely from government sources and from parental fees for service. If either or both dry up, the operation goes out of business very quickly. Unlike many other commercial enterprises, childcare and kindergarten enterprises are small, and have to be sufficiently fluid, in both management and delivery of services, for change to be effected with minimum fuss and within a short time frame.

As many of the better-run childcare centres, particularly the good-quality ones, have a cooperative style of management structure where decisions are cooperatively agreed to, organisational resistance is less of a problem. However, this does not imply that change in early childhood establishments is without its inherent insecurities—for staff, for management and for the parents (clients).

If you consider each of the factors of resistance to change presented in Table 2.1 you will see the complexity of such resistance. Some of these factors are relevant to early childhood services and relevant to change processes, others might be more appropriate to larger business enterprises. It is important to keep in mind that early childhood services deal with the 'non-compulsory' sector of human and social services and, hence, depend on 'clients' for their very existence. Child care and kindergarten to a lesser but still realistic extent are commercial enterprises, no matter what their management structure. Some of the factors listed in Table 2.1 under organisational sources are, therefore, appropriate for consideration in early childhood management.

PLANNING FOR CHANGE

The most effective change in any organisation is the change that has been planned. Of course, the sequence in planning, as indeed the strategy of the plan itself, will vary according to the complexity of the proposed change and the size of the organisation affected by the change. Most planned change, however, has the following six steps in the process:

1. recognition that there is a performance gap;
2. recognition that there is a need for change and diagnosis of the problem;
3. creation of a climate for effective change;
4. consideration of and selection of possible strategies for overcoming the problem;
5. implementation of the chosen strategies; and
6. evaluation of the effectiveness of the change.

These steps represent a simplified strategy for implementing change. They say nothing about the timeline for change in the strategy. This factor also depends on the complexity of the change and the size of the organisation. In education, for example, there would be a different timeline if the change were merely mechanical, such as moving a system's headquarters from one location to another, from the one employed if the change were as complex as introducing a new curriculum framework throughout the whole schooling system.

The six steps in the simplified change process illustrated above could entail the following.

Performance gap

A recognition by teachers and caregivers that things could be done more efficiently and with better outcomes, *or* the realisation by systems managers that there was too great a difference in the performance of the staff working within the system and hence too great a difference in outcomes across the system. This latter example could relate to curriculum, evaluation procedures and the like.

Need for change and diagnosis of the problem

Having realised that there was a gap in the overall performance of the organisation, all parties involved, including management, would agree that there was some need for change and attempt to clarify the exact problem and how the problem might be overcome. For example, an education system might find that the variations in student results at some common examination/evaluation were so great that they were causing some embarrassment within the system and concern among parents. Or, at a more basic level, the staff of a kindergarten or childcare centre might be concerned that their method of daily and weekly planning was overlooking important elements in the children's development and believe that a system of evaluation based on child observations using a particular proforma could assist in overcoming the problem.

Creating a climate for change

This could entail regular workshops or discussions about the concerns raised and the needs evident in an attempt to get the people in the change process on-side, thus eliminating or at least lessening any potential resistance to change. The purpose of this step is to get total support for the proposed change. For example, where staff in a kindergarten or childcare centre are being challenged to review their practices of program planning and where some staff are resisting the proposed changes, daily assistance in the planning by a team leader who could highlight the problems in the existing system as they arise might win over reluctant staff to the idea of pursuing the proposed changes.

Selecting strategies for the proposed change

Here the persons responsible for the change process, together with the staff involved (and in the case of education and child care—the parents), consider all the implications relating to the identified performance gap and the possible solutions for overcoming this gap. Such implications could include matters of finance, changes to textbooks or the balance between the subjects in a curriculum and freeing staff time for planning. In early childhood situations it could mean all of those mentioned plus parental input and maybe some external assistance with new ways of programming. In all cases the benefits of the change proposed should be highlighted.

Implementation of the selected change process

This step implies that the process is generally agreed on, that the people in the process are cognisant of the aims and objectives and the timeline for the process, and that they are willing to try out the innovations that come with the new procedures. As indicated before, depending on the magnitude of the change underway, the timeline agreed to should be such that implementation is possible—that there is a degree of flexibility in the time scheduled for the various stages in the implementation plan (yet not so flexible that it could be a never-ending saga). In childcare establishments, it is often the case that external assistance is sought to work with the centre personnel throughout the change process. This assistance is valuable when, for example, care centres work on upgrading the quality of their care for accreditation or other reasons. The Australian federal government has funded the various state Lady Gowrie Child Centres to provide resources and assistance to childcare centres. Similarly, the various state licensing authorities provide an advisory service to early childhood organisations on matters relating to licensing requirements (e.g. building requirements and curriculum).

Fullan (1982; 1992) enumerates a number of factors that affect implementation, namely:

1. **Characteristics of the change**
   - need and relevance of the change
   - clarity
   - complexity
   - quality and practicality of program (materials etc.).
2. **Characteristics at the school district level**
   - the history of innovative attempts
   - the adoption process
   - central administration support and involvement
   - staff development (in-service) and participation
   - timeline and information system (evaluation)
   - board and community characteristics.
3. **Characteristics at the school level**
   - the principal
   - teacher–teacher relations
   - teacher characteristics and orientations.

4. **Characteristics external to the local system**
   - role of government
   - external assistance.

Evaluation

This important step is sometimes seen as the end of the change process, but it really is not. The change process is a continuous one, cyclical in nature, as once an element of change has been achieved other areas in the organisation where change is desirable come to the forefront of attention. It is necessary for the organisation to evaluate whether the performance gap initially recognised by the people in the organisation has been reduced and whether or not the change strategy was successful, and by how much. This step is also diagnostic, in that the evaluation done can be diagnosed to see where successes were achieved and where improvements or further changes in the ensuing process could be made.

There are three general strategies for organisational change, namely:

1. the structural approach, where the change is related to an organisation's structure such as changing departments, roles and responsibilities of staff;
2. the technological approach, where the change is related to the technologies of the workplace (e.g. the introduction of computers and computer systems into management). Here the change relates to how jobs are done;
3. the people-centred approaches, where the changes are aimed at improving employee skills and attitudes. Individual change strategies were introduced by Kurt Lewin in the 1930s and later developed by Schein in the 1960s. They came up with a model that had four steps—
   - desire for change,
   - unfreezing (where a person is motivated to at least attempt to change),
   - changing (where a person is presented with new patterns of behaviour/methods etc. and adopts them), and
   - refreezing (where the changed attitudes, skills etc. are incorporated into the individual's normal pattern of behaviour).

Case study 2.2 takes many of the elements raised in this chapter—change, change management, processes of change—and shows how these can occur using a systems approach.

Case study 2.2
Planning for change—a systems approach

SACSA (South Australian Curriculum, Standards and Accountability) was the outcome of considerable planning and thought over a period of time, and relates to substantial curriculum change in South Australia. Curriculum change is a never-ending activity and is generally stimulated by the need for educational establishments to keep abreast of the rapidly changing social environment, itself stimulated by advances in technology, research, social conditions and the general knowledge explosion existing in dynamic societies. In the case of South Australia the stimulus came also from educators who could see the need for change.

Prior curriculum documents and processes for implementing curricula in South Australia are detailed in two curriculum documents: Foundation Areas of Learning (Department for Education and Children's Services, DECS 1996), which relates to the preschool years, and Curriculum Statements and Profiles (Curriculum Corporation 1993), which relates to the compulsory years of schooling. While these documents were still considered relevant and promulgated the strategy of curriculum outcomes, it was considered timely in the latter half of the 1990s to review school curricula, and particularly to consider the desirability of a curriculum framework that would encompass the early childhood years through to the end of schooling (Year 12) in an integrated and continuous design.

As a result, a vision and values statement was prepared by the Department of Education, Training and Employment (DETE) South Australia entitled *Foundations for the Future* (DECS 1997) and was issued in 1997. Stehn (1999) said that this statement emerged from a major consultation that canvassed the opinions and expectations of students, parents, educators and community members across the state. Here we can see the beginnings of the planning for change. This consultation represented the recognition stage in the planning cycle described above.

The document *Foundations for the Future* also detailed the values that the people of the state could expect from any curricula designed for the children of the state. These values included trust, honesty, integrity, responsibility, equity, fairness, diligence and excellence. Five strategic directions for public education and care to the year 2010 were described. The discussion period took some two years and culminated in an unpublished document entitled 'Leading in Learning', which set the underlying philosophy and direction for SACSA.

A detailed account of the South Australian Curriculum, Standards and Accountability Framework (SACSA 2001) can be obtained on http://www.sacsa.sa.edu.au

In Case study 2.2 we see the developments of the process leading to steps 2 and 3 of the change process enumerated earlier. No two processes are exactly the same and there is often a blurring of the steps in the process. Once the momentum for change is established, the actual change process agreed to can be as swift or as slow as desired by the orchestrators of the change.

Outcomes of the discussions and consultations during the years 1997/98 centred on the areas of DETE 1999, cited in Stehn 1999: 2:

- making the language of the documents more accessible and user-friendly;
- using language consistently across the learning areas and in each learning area;
- reducing the volume of the documents;
- eliminating, or identifying, as a support for integrated planning, the overlap across areas of learning; and
- improving the connections between the Statements and Profiles and other curriculum directions.

Such considerations led to decisions on the possible design of the new curricula. As the existing Framework models were working quite well, it was decided that the new design would also be in the form of a Framework document rather than a prescriptive design of content and teaching/learning methodology. It represented the base structure around which the schools and children's services could build their curricula. In addition, a number of committees were established to oversee the preparation of the Framework, and the writing process began with a contract being awarded after open advertisement. Here, the process reached step 4 as described in the change process noted above.

Details of the Framework are available on the Web. Suffice it to say here that SACSA became one cohesive framework based on an assumption of the integration of curriculum planning, teaching, learning, assessment and reporting for the years from birth to Year 12.

Implementation of the chosen strategies (step 5) included the preparation of an implementation plan and material essential to explain to the educators in the field what was required. The plan indicated that implementing SACSA was departmental priority for 2001 and 2002, and detailed how this would be achieved so that by the end of 2002 all sites and services would report to their communities about learners' achievements in relation to the Curriculum Standards in the SACSA Framework (SACSA Implementation Plan 2001–2002: 11).

The plan indicated how the responsibility for implementing SACSA would be a shared responsibility of all site, district and state office leaders. A SACSA Implementing Steering Committee would oversee and coordinate implementation activities at state and district levels and provide direction for an external evaluation of the implementation process.

Support for the Framework's implementation came in the form of appropriate printed material, which included guides, tasks, news and feedback information, professional development tools and activities, and sharing of ideas and resources. Important material supporting the curriculum account-

Table 2.2 Initial key dates and actions in the development of the SACSA Framework

Time frame	Action
Terms 1–3, 2000	Trialling of the Framework in selected sites
Term 4, 2000	Final draft of the trial forwarded to the chief executive of the department for approval
November 2000	Approval of the SACSA Framework final draft posted on SACSA website
December 2000	Implementation plan distributed to all sites
January 2001	Sets of the Framework distributed to all sites, and site leaders provided with details for ordering material
March 2001	New interactive SACSA website on-line materials ordered for each site
April 2001	Distribution of printed material ordered
Terms 1 and 2, 2001	Leader of professional development program and activities to support program implementation

Source: DETE (1998).

ability process was also available and included moderated assessment tasks. As indicated in Table 2.2, a variety of professional development activities were planned for site leaders to enable them to understand the purposes, goals and processes of the Framework and to act as a support network.

So began the Implementation Plan. What is included here is only the beginning of implementing the SACSA Framework. The plan included activities for two years and an evaluation.

Professional development was also part of the Implementation Plan, and the timeline for a development program covered all of 2001 and 2002. In relation to professional development, the plan aimed: to be responsive to the varying needs of leaders and educators across South Australia; to be flexible according to local requirements and issues; and to result in practical outcomes that could be shared with other educators. Professional development included site-based activities utilising allocated professional development time. The plan also included professional development for leaders; for strategic district activities, local and statewide professional networks; and other support from departmental sources.

Evaluation is the final step in the process of planned change. In the case of SACSA the evaluation process at the initial design stage covered the trial step of the Framework's implementation and was done during January–April 2001 by the contracted evaluators—The Curriculum Corporation. The full report is available on the SACSA website. The executive summary commented on the process of evaluation within the terms of reference.

The summary of the evaluation findings included such comments as:

- The process used delivered the product to sites within the timeline planned.
- The process used was seen by participants to have many benefits and had a positive impact on what was achieved and how it was achieved.
- The levels of professional debate and scrutiny generated through the processes were seen to contribute to a more robust and defensible curriculum.
- Many of the respondents saw powerful benefits gained through the partnerships that were established.
- The consultation process used to conceptualise and shape the Framework was valued by most respondents.
- The project intention was the development of one Framework. There is evidence of tension between these elements.

These are but a few of the evaluation findings. They indicate how the evaluation of the process of the trial stage could assist in the refining of the processes of the Implementation Plan as well as, by inference, any glaring problems that might arise in relation to the Framework proper.

At the time of writing this chapter the SACSA Implementation Committee is preparing a plan for the evaluation of the implementation process. It will be published on the Web when completed and it will be clear as to how the various bands (including the 'early years band') are separately evaluated. In conjunction with the planned evaluation, other forms of evaluation will be carried out, such as the one being done for from birth to 3 years of the early years band. This particular evaluation has been funded by a federal government 'Strategic Partnerships with Industry, Research and Training' (SPIRT) grant and is attempting to see whether the curriculum framework makes any difference to the quality of the work of childcare centres in their planning for infant and toddler groups.

LEADERSHIP DURING CHANGE

'Leading is empowering.' Such a statement implies that the effective leader in education is one who builds up the professional's self-perception as being empowered (Rodd 1997: 4). Empowerment, in the sense that we are using it in the context of change, is as Stone (1995: 294) implied: practising professionals taking ownership and accepting their right to be involved in deciding about and influencing change.

The topic of leadership has been dealt with fully in Chapter 1. It is important here, however, that some consideration be given to the role of the leader in the change process. Here we see the leader as a shape-changer whose role and work shifts constantly according to need (Razik & Swanson 2001: 48).

What Case study 2.2 on implementing the SACSA Framework has shown clearly is that strong leadership at all levels of implementing change is essential to successful implementation. This is why the SACSA Implementation Plan had a major component on professional development, including professional development for leaders.

Leadership during the process of change is a complex activity. In some ways it can be likened to leading a cultural change, as education in the form of pre-schooling has, over the years, generated its own 'culture'. Certainly when we talk of schooling as a process we get into the realm of people's feelings, thoughts and actions. There are assumptions about education (rightly conceived or not), about curricula, about the processes of teaching and learning. These assumptions are coupled to internal integration and external adaptation, to form, in this case, an educational culture. Schein (1985: 2) claims that creating, managing and sometimes restructuring organisational culture are some of the most decisive functions of leadership:

- *We have already commented that change is always with us. In education, environmental conditions are constantly changing and therefore the leaders in education must keep up with this change and be able to manipulate 'the educational culture' to ensure that the organisation survives, indeed thrives as a result of the change required.*
- *The leader, therefore, must be well informed of the changing processes being implemented at any particular time as well as have a global view of where the process will lead eventually. The leader must act from information gained from a wide band of interests surveyed and not a narrow one.*
- *The leader in the change process is very much like the director of a dramatic play. If the director wants to get the best out of the performers then he/she must lead these performers to 'see' things differently if the production is to remain a unified activity. It could very easily not become the sum of its parts especially if the direction of the production is unclear and not a shared one.*

So it is in education and care environments. While direction can often be established as a result of collective negotiation, unity in purpose and direction generally rests with the producer/leader. Success in most things in management depends on the balance between being told what to do and being encouraged to participate in resolving the best way of doing something. One way may save time, but not necessarily so. The other way may take more time to find the right direction but be achieved more quickly and efficiently, as unity in purpose has thus been achieved.

The SACSA Framework implementation model described earlier places a lot of responsibility on the leader(s) involved, but not to the exclusion of everyone else involved in the process. In some ways the process empowers all staff, particularly those teaching at the classroom level: after all, it is at this level that the greatest change is directed. The people involved at all levels are expected to take their share of responsibility for the implementation strategies. The 'leaders' are seen more as resource persons and communicators with the knowledge of the wider implications of the total process being implemented, rather than as those with the 'vision' and authority that comes with superior knowledge and position. However, a knowledge base is essential for leadership.

What, then, is the knowledge base that an effective leader in early childhood needs to have in order to facilitate effective change in early childhood centres? First, the leader needs to accept that:

- Change is inevitable.
- Change can be perceived to be positive, negative, or have elements of both.
- Enforced change is more difficult to implement than change that people have identified as needed, and planned in advance.
- Change can be very threatening if it is not understood and may create resistance, particularly among the more insecure staff.
- Change is a process.
- Some staff will be good change agents and able to help others to understand and accept change.
- Support must be given readily to staff so that the change process is not alienating.
- The change process ought to be a team approach.
- To effect successful change takes time, and allowing adequate time is a fundamental ingredient of the total process.
- Effective change can increase the autonomy of staff and empower them as professionals.
- Effective communication is central to any change.

What we are saying here is that in times of educational change, and particularly during the period of planned change, the role of the leader is crucial in successfully achieving the desired change. However, leadership need not be a factor of management hierarchy because, as discussed in Chapter 1, managers are not necessarily leaders. Leadership should happen at all levels within an organisation, and in educational establishments this includes the classroom teachers. Where all people involved in the change process are empowered with a sense of responsibility as well as commitment to the direction of the change being implemented, a more effective, cooperative form of leadership will be established. This kind of leadership shifts the balance in planning towards the personal, negotiated and empowering side, rather than being the outcome of some hierarchical activity.

ADOPTING CHANGE

Fullan (1982) stated in an earlier publication that there are specific factors that affect whether or not a change is adopted. These are:

- existence and quality of innovations;
- access to information;
- advocacy from central administrators;
- teacher pressure/support;
- consultants and change agents;
- community pressure/support/apathy/opposition;
- availability of federal or other funds;
- new central legislation or policy (federal/state/provincial);
- problem-solving incentives for adoption; and
- bureaucratic incentives for adoption.

Fullan and Hargreaves (1992) believe strongly that educational change is not a single entity. It is, to a certain extent, multidimensional. Teachers may implement some, all or none of the change dimensions. Change in practice may be very different from change in theory.

Where we have systemic change (such as that adopted by state governments, departments of education or religious school systems), there is a known acceptance of the change by the authoritative elements of the system. However, while this acceptance is in one sense comforting to teachers, it can cause problems if the 'system' also does not accept that there are wide differences among and between schools forming the system. Concentrating too rigidly on 'outcomes' may be detrimental to the effective implementation of any curriculum change.

Movements that require preschool curricula to lead on to primary school curricula may have their advantages but also have potential disadvantages. Some people might think that having a mandated curriculum for 'before school' requires the preschool teacher to get the children 'ready' for school in a certain way. It could also be seen as a 'downward push' in the curriculum requirements and standards to be achieved. This may be so, but it need not be so.

Having a curriculum that is sufficiently flexible yet with clearly articulated goals and objectives can only help all early childhood teachers and caregivers. If it is well developed, such a curriculum can guide the teacher's planning for outcomes that are developmentally appropriate. While it cannot be said that in the past preschool education was devoid of a curriculum, in many cases it was not presented in such a way that it could be defended as educationally and developmentally sound.

PUTTING CHANGE INTO DAILY PRACTICE

So far in this chapter we have been exploring the idea that change is all about us, part of our everyday experiences, and affects all areas of early childhood services. Here we look more directly at how change in its many forms affects the daily operations of childcare centres and other early childhood services.

Schrag, Nelson and Siminowsky (1998) in Neugebauer and Neugebauer (1998: 232) gave three examples of change that affected early childhood centres on a daily basis. First, the problems associated with the addition of a new room for infants in an operating childcare centre are described. While the addition of the new service was successful in that it was oversubscribed, there were problems generated because of this action which affected the other elements of the centre's work. The staff were upset because equipment and funding were reduced to support the new activity, and the centre's director's time as support was directed away from the existing service to the new one.

The second example related to the employment of a new head teacher in a kindergarten. The existing staff were not considered for promotion to the position and were threatened by the new ideas and enthusiasm of the new head teacher. The third example related to the introduction of computers into an after-school-hours program. The teachers were threatened as they were not proficient with computers, and the obvious enthusiasm of the children added to the stress caused by this curriculum innovation.

These are fairly common examples of change in early childhood settings. The chapter by Schrag et al. in Neugebauer and Neugebauer (1998) goes on to discuss how effective leaders can help staff overcome the problems generated by such change, such as through building up staff to be resilient, keeping staff informed, providing support and, above all, involving staff in the change process.

We cannot get away from the very important role of the leader in resolving any change, be it minor or major in degree. In early childhood settings the leader is usually the centre's director or, in large centres where there are teams operating, the elected or nominated team leader. Such leaders have to get the job done, and this involves managing staff and children (inasmuch as the children's activities are the product of the staff's planning), organising equipment and material, meeting parents, and liaison with senior management. However, in all these tasks it is the management and leadership of staff that represents the major activity of the leader. In many cases it is the leader who is the buffer between competing pressures in the change process.

Obviously, when change is present the leader has to be well informed of the direction in which the change is headed. Mentoring staff is crucial: it is not enough for staff simply to be involved in the process of change—they often need help in implementing the change. The leader has to structure such mentoring activities into her/his daily work plan. Very often it is done 'on top of' all the other, normal, activities of the leader.

The second example given at the beginning of this section—that of the new staff member, alive and enthusiastic and a threat to existing staff—poses another problem for the leader and management. Certainly the change in such situations is threatening to some of the existing staff who may, over time, come to accept the new person but in the short term have to accommodate him/her within the total centre operation. In the hands of a skilled leader/manager the skills and enthusiasm of the new staff member can assist in the building up of the staff's expertise. However, the new staff member must first be accepted by the old staff.

The amount and degree of change to the existing practices of an early childhood centre that happen on a daily basis are too great to do justice to here. Most managers and leaders can cope with situations that generate regular change, such as the absence of staff, by having routines to overcome them (e.g. relief staff lists with easy routines for telephone contact). Other changes that relate to implementing new curricula or adding a new service within existing resources, such as the first example given at the beginning of this section, are not so easy to manage. There is no one 'recipe' for managing change, as each change situation is different from any other simply because the people are different. What is crucial is the capacity of the staff to accommodate change when it occurs, even to anticipate it, and certainly to direct it. The important element here is staff development.

Some people have the ability to adapt to change, others do not. Schrag, Nelson and Siminowsky (1998, in Neugebauer & Neugebauer 1998: 235) proposed that there were five attitudes shared by those who are best able to deal with change, namely:

1. challenge—an openness to change;
2. commitment—a high degree of involvement in what one is doing;
3. control—a sense of personal impact on external change;
4. confidence—the recognition that no situation puts your personal worth on the line;
5. connection—the extent of interpenetration you are willing to establish between yourself, others and your environment. Interaction with the external environment, or making connections, somehow appears to allow a parallel process to take place internally, enabling a person to develop an increasingly sophisticated system of adaptability to change.

One other element to daily change practices is the importance of networking for support. In early childhood, as the centres providing the service and the families requiring the service are in reasonably close contact, parental understanding and support in change processes are desirable and usually helpful. Situations such as where the outside environment needs major or minor renovating can be facilitated with the support, including physical labour, of parent groups. Similarly, other external agencies—such as health and welfare agencies—can assist an early childhood centre by collaborating in the change process. Such support may be crucial when, for example, adding a particular service directed at children with special needs. Other professional, union or social service groups can also be supports during the process of change and should be co-opted into the process when appropriate. Every successful early childhood centre has a network of support groups and agencies on which they can call when needed.

Case study 2.3
Change instigated by a classroom teacher

A teacher of a kindergarten 1 class in a small, private early childhood centre in Singapore was concerned that the recently introduced government policies for early childhood in Singapore were not being heeded by teachers generally and were misunderstood by parents. She decided to experiment with the curriculum for her class of children by introducing the project approach as central to her curriculum.

The two main reasons for her desire to experiment with curriculum change were first, as mentioned above, to see whether the overly teacher-directed curriculum in kindergartens could be modified while still covering requirements in the government-set curriculum; second, to see whether the projects that the children would embrace could be less of the 'academic/cognitive' nature favoured in schools in Singapore and more of the kind following the interests of the children while still covering the 'required' academic content of the curriculum. She wanted, in essence, to identify the strengths and weaknesses of the project approach for the individual development of the children.

The research project lasted for eight weeks. The children chosen for the project attended the kindergarten for the whole day. They worked on the projects in the afternoons after completing their normal 'academic' work in the mornings. This arrangement allowed the teacher to compare the outcomes of the two teaching methods on the same children.

Two projects were attempted during the eight-week period. The first was a result of construction work on an adjacent building block, and turned into a 'construction machine project'. The second was a project on musical instruments, following an episode when one child brought his violin to the kindergarten to show his friends. During the two projects the children were involved in activities covering creative development; knowledge and understanding of the world; mathematics; language and literacy; personal and social development; and physical development.

The findings can be summarised as follows:

- Once children realised they were allowed to initiate their own activities, they did so with enthusiasm.
- The project approach extended the children's learning and added a new focus to their activities: the children became proficient at extending their ideas and questions.
- There was an increase in motivation present even for those activities that were of an 'academic' nature (as evidenced on the recorded observations): the children used their knowledge to acquire new information.

Continued

- The project approach did not diminish the 'traditional' academic work the children had to be involved with.
- The children became more independent, and with some children this independence was transferred to other areas of school life.
- All developmental areas could be included and extended: the wide variety of activities engaged in enabled this to happen.

Used with the permission of Tracy Bennet 2001, Singapore

Observations that can be made regarding Case study 2.3:

- Traditional methods could highlight the limitations of the teacher, not the ability of the children.
- The project approach should not be the only curriculum method used at any one time. There could be a problem with large classes.
- It is the teacher's responsibility to balance the curriculum, not the children's: for example, children might initiate too many 'creative' activities to the detriment of other activities.

Self-assessment exercise

Students should attempt the following self-assessment task. Coming from Steers and Black (1994: 678), it focuses on a person's receptivity to change. There are no correct or incorrect answers—differences across people are natural.

Instructions

For each of the items listed below, select the answer that best suits your degree of agreement or disagreement. When you are finished, add up your total points.

	1	2	3	4	5	
Strongly agree						**Strongly disagree**

1. I continually like to try new things.
   1   2   3   4   5

2. I would prefer to have a job that forces me to learn new skills regularly.
   1   2   3   4   5

3. I like things just the way they are in my life.
   1   2   3   4   5

4. Life to me is just one new adventure after another.
   1   2   3   4   5

5. For the past several years I have known exactly what I want to do with my life.
   1   2   3   4   5

6. I like to keep all of my things in their proper place.
   1   2   3   4   5

7. My ideal job has clear, fixed requirements that I can count on.
   1   2   3   4   5

8. My friends often tell me that I am adventuresome.
   1   2   3   4   5

9. I see myself changing jobs and careers fairly often in my life.
   1   2   3   4   5

10. I get bored doing the same things over and over.
   1   2   3   4   5

Now, add up your score and consider the following categories:

- A score of 10–20 indicates high receptivity to change.
- A score of 21–39 indicates a modest receptivity to change.
- A score of 40–50 indicates a low receptivity to change.

When you have completed your self-assessment, consider how you might improve your abilities as a leader in early childhood.

CHAPTER SUMMARY

This chapter has attempted to deal with the process of change in early childhood settings.

- Change is, more or less, the only certainty in the management of services, including those in the broad field of early childhood.
- Change is not something to be feared by organisations; rather, it should be seen as a challenge if organisations are to remain viable in an ever-changing environment.
- Renewal and change processes are mandatory for survival and effectiveness.
- The chapter included some thoughts on the theory of change and in particular systems theory, as we work in systems, large or small, and what affects one part of a system affects all in one way or other.

- The process of change in the various early childhood workplaces was considered under a number of headings, as change in early childhood is dynamic, often far-reaching, often disturbing to staff and management, and seemingly never-ending.
- Resistance to change was considered in the light of staff behaviour and, from a leadership point of view, in the light of staff development.
- The roles and responsibilities of management and leadership in the change process were also considered.
- Three case studies showed various ways of coping with change in very diverse contexts.
- Finally, the chapter outlined the day-to-day changes that have had to be dealt with by management so as to keep the services operating.

 Discussion and reflection

1. Identify and discuss one major change which you as a professional have confronted.

    (a)   Who assisted you to cope with the change process?
    (b)   How successful was the outcome of this change?
    (c)   Write down one way that you think a manager of an organisation undergoing a major change could show positive concern for his/her staff.
    (d)   Ask a work colleague to describe a change she/he went through. Was it positive or negative? Why?

2. 'Organisations are made up of groups of people working together to achieve common goals.' Reflect on what this very important statement means in relation to early childhood centres. Also, consider what the common goals might be for early childhood centres.

3. Discuss what the terms 'open system' and 'closed system' might mean in your own early childhood centre or in one that you know. Go to the dictionary to find out the meaning of the terms interrelationship, interaction, and interdependence. Write down the differences between these important terms.

4. Discuss this statement: 'Education leads change'.

    (a)   Do you agree or disagree with it?
    (b)   Try to think of a case you know of where education did lead to a significant change. Was it an exciting outcome? Was it futures-oriented?

5. What changes in early childhood, if any, are you aware of in other countries?

    (a)   How dramatic have these changes been?
    (b)   In what ways have early childhood services changed? For example, has availability of services improved? Has quality of provision improved?

6. Write down some names (labels) which describe early childhood centres/schools in your town, state or country.

   (a) Have these names changed during your professional life? If so, why?
   (b) Write down the qualifications now needed to teach in early childhood contexts in your town, state or country. How have these requirements changed over the years? Why is this so?

7. Why is it that the term 'industry' is unpopular with many professionals? What are your own views about this term? Are there other terms that might be more acceptable?

8. Think about the current status of early childhood professionals throughout the world.

   (a) Are these professionals held in high or low esteem in your country? Why is this so?
   (b) What changes would you like to see occurring in relation to the points made?

Chapter **3**

Leadership practices for effective partnerships with families

Learning to work effectively with families with young children is a cornerstone of everyday practice for early childhood professionals around the world. Yet it is also one of the most complex and complicated dimensions of professional practice encountered in centre administration, management and leadership in early childhood. An analysis is made here of the changing nature of families and the importance of adapting professional practices to suit complex contexts, especially in respecting and responding to diversity. Excerpts of conversations with leading early childhood practitioners in Australia and in Singapore illustrate new ways of dealing with recurrent dilemmas when working with families.

Outcomes

At the conclusion of this chapter, the reader should have:

- developed an appreciation of respecting and responding to family diversity;
- acquired an understanding of the importance of values in guiding interactions with families;
- recognised the changing nature of families and the need to adjust professional practices accordingly;
- an understanding of the differing roles and responsibilities of parents and professionals;
- recognised the importance of continuing professional training to update knowledge and skills pertaining to working with families;
- developed an appreciation of early childhood leadership in bringing together divergent perspectives to respond effectively to children and their families.

RESPECTING AND RESPONDING TO DIVERSITY

Having examined a range of international studies on school–family–community partnerships, Epstein and Sanders (1998: 392) concluded that 'parents everywhere love and care for their children and they want to be involved in all aspects of their children's development, including their education'. Working with families requires early childhood professionals to take account of the social diversity of their local community, and this may or may not be fully reflected in their programs. Where social diversity is present it means respectful consideration of child and family variations, such as family structure and size, parents' marital and employment status, lifestyles, ethnicity and religion. Community perceptions about the best way to bring up a child can convey conflicting messages due to differing beliefs, attitudes and values. Shimoni and Baxter (1996) take the reader through a variety of scenarios, developed from the point of view of parents and professionals, which explore factors that hinder effective collaboration, including preconceived ideas, differences in status and power, differing world views and unclear policies. Such examples serve to illustrate the complexity of promoting and developing effective communication channels with families using early childhood services.

Diversity in early childhood is also reflected in the nature of issues that early childhood professionals are required to consider in their provision of services to families. Bhavangari and Gonzalez-Mena (1997), for instance, discuss particular concerns of cultural diversity with regard to the care of infants and toddlers. Butterworth and Candy (1998) as well as Ebbeck and Glover (1998) have explored the perspectives of working with families from particular indigenous communities and immigrant backgrounds respectively. Likewise, special thematic editions of journals such as the *Australian Journal of Early Childhood* have been dedicated to the examination of issues pertaining to working with children who have additional needs, in particular children with social-emotional, physical and intellectual disabilities. The challenges of working with children who have experienced trauma as refugees and asylum seekers have been the focus of study for educators such as Palmer (2000) and Waniganayake (2001). Collaboration with parents over curriculum matters has been addressed by writers such as Carter (2000) and Fleer (1996). More recently, emergent literacy research is putting the spotlight on re-examining home–school connections (e.g. see Ashton & Cairney 2001; Jayatilaka 2001; Raban 2001). In Australia, these interests have also been linked to research on school readiness and starting-school matters (e.g. see Meredith, Perry, Borg & Dockett 1999; de Lemos & Mellor 1994). Taken together, such studies reflect the breadth and depth of the nature of parent–staff interactions in early childhood.

Fleet and Clyde (1993: 18) identified five key characteristics of effective partnerships in early childhood, as follows:

1. respect for everyone involved;
2. courteous and open two-way communication, which includes sharing information;
3. frank, positive and constructive approaches to problem solving by everyone;
4. opportunities to make genuine contributions to the project or service; and
5. ongoing interaction among all.

These characteristics are based on respecting diversity, and provide a principle-based approach to working with families in early childhood services. In contrast, the adoption of a more regulatory approach with prescriptive guidelines to manage parent–staff communications when using children's services is not recommended. Tightly defined provisions can obstruct and deter the start-up of social interactions, and emotive imperatives about children's wellbeing can exacerbate communication difficulties for both parents and professionals.

It is now more than two decades since Bronfenbrenner's ecological theory of human development (1979) gained prominence in designing and developing early childhood programs and later provided a framework for government policies (Bronfenbrenner & Weiss 1983). During the 1980s worsening economic conditions in Western industrialised nations such as Australia and the USA required governments, unions and corporations alike to consider ways of restructuring the economy. During this era, as a way of supporting employees with young children, 'family-friendly' workplace policies (Adam 1991; Biggs 1989; Vesk 1989) were launched. The establishment and growth of employer-sponsored childcare centres by large organisations such as hospitals and banks, and by major corporations such as Erickson in Sweden, are developments stemming from these policy initiatives. In Australia, the federal government, through the provision of significant financial incentives including interest-free loans and tax exemptions to employers embracing childcare provision, overtly supported these initiatives (Brenann 1998a). In addition, support was given through various benefits available to employees with family responsibilities, including flexible working hours, income supplements and parental leave provisions (Kamerman & Kahn 1987; Seyler, Monro & Garand 1995; Wolcott 1991). Much of the childcare benefits to corporations have now all but disappeared, though the commitment to remain family-friendly is retained within the overall policy frameworks by both government and corporate employers. With declining birthrates in industrially affluent countries such as Australia and Singapore, parental leave options are now attracting the attention of both the public and the government (Goward 2002).

External as well as internal forces emanating from the operational context of children's services can also influence parent–staff interactions during early childhood. External sources experienced by families include the pressure of balancing work and family responsibilities. Implementation of centre policies, such as when a child is mildly ill, can at times present a dilemma for both staff and parents. The parent rushing off to work who is told that the centre cannot accept the child can have difficulty finding alternative care at such short notice. Here, a single incident or exchange between staff and parents can alter the dynamics of the relationship either positively or negatively. Keeping the partnership alive, therefore, relies heavily on individuals' commitment to staying in touch, being flexible, and seeking peaceful resolutions to problems as they arise. Research is scarce on topics such as the care of children when they are not well. Some avenues for consideration are presented in the following excerpt by Barbara Donegan from Australia, who discusses her views on responding to families when their children are unwell.

Responding to families when children are unwell

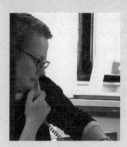

BARBARA DONEGAN
Director
John Street Community Early Childhood Co-operative
Melbourne, Australia

1. What are some of the complexities that early childhood professionals face in responding to children when they are not well?

Lots of childhood illnesses start off with very similar symptoms like a runny nose etc. which then may or (more often) may not go on to something more definable. Therefore, when a child is unwell it can be difficult to know immediately what you are dealing with. Early childhood professionals working in child care or preschools get a lot of experience with unwell children. In addition to considering the risks to other children and staff, we have to be practical about the level of care we can offer at the centre when a child is ill. For example, if the child needs one-on-one care, we realistically can't offer that; so child care is not the place for that child to be that day.

Another issue is that you are dealing mostly with working parents, sometimes without local family or other support. When their children are unwell, these parents have the added pressures of balancing work and family responsibilities. For parents and childcare staff this means determining exactly when 'unwell' means not well enough to be at child care. There is a need for understanding the pressures that families are under and building trust with families so that staff

Continued

will make well-considered decisions at this stage. For childcare staff who are not trained health professionals, there is a need to have a practical set of guidelines to operate by when determining what constitutes being well enough to be in child care and what doesn't. Such guidelines should be readily observable by parents and staff. We are also mindful that children can and will get mild colds and coughs. Having said this, we can appreciate that parents will need on occasion to leave a mildly unwell child with us, due to work pressure.

At my centre, with the help of a parent with medical training we have developed a set of clear criteria for assessing wellness in children. So we can look at the overall picture of the child in deciding not only when they are not well enough to attend but also when they are not unwell enough to warrant going home. I think also that if your focus is on assessing wellness as well as illness, then you have set up a climate for communication that is more inclusive and more supportive of parents but also more meaningful for all families.

2. You were trained as a nurse before you became an early childhood professional. What has having this dual professional background meant to you in practice?

Being a nurse is a really good background for early childhood work. It gives you an understanding about the physiology and the practicalities of illness in children's services. Strangely, it can (and did, in my case) provide a poor orientation for the more day-to-day childhood illnesses that present in child care, because these children don't come into hospitals. When I first started in child care, the more experienced early childhood staff knew a lot more about what a measles or chickenpox rash looked like than I did! My nursing background has been very handy for reviewing and updating accident and medication records and other paperwork associated with health things. It's also good as backup support for staff, who are able to get me to double-check on things—for example when there are day-to-day accidents such as a bump on a head or perhaps a query to do with giving medication. It has also been good for developing and reviewing health policies for the centre. These are reviewed by me, as well as by parents with medical and health backgrounds, to ensure that our policies are up-to-date, relevant and practical. It can also be very handy for understanding the medical backgrounds of children who may have something of note prior to or since commencing child care.

3. Today there is a lot of concern about the impact of child illnesses on early childhood staff health and wellbeing. As centre director, how do you handle this concern?

You certainly need to look at the complexities of balancing child and family needs. However, while being mindful of family pressure, we must also ensure that staff are supported. Child care is a very busy and challenging job even with healthy children, so we need to be realistic about what we can expect of staff in relation to an unwell child. Of course this really boils down to good communication with families.

You have to also encourage staff to be responsible for their own wellbeing—recognising their own symptoms: if they are unwell, they too must stay at home.

Continued

And staff need to be supported to consider their own workloads. If there is a continuous pattern of illnesses, then we need to look at work routines and structures to see whether these can be changed. Then there is the possibility of funding immunisation costs for all staff, or at least providing information on immunisations with encouragement to update them. This goes a long way to ensuring that staff feel valued, and that there is recognition of the complexity of the responsibilities of their role.

4. Under what circumstances would you accept a child with a chronic illness?

We believe that child care is a valuable experience for children, so we would certainly want to extend this opportunity to *all* children, including those with chronic illness. There are enormous variations in chronic illness. For example, children who have insulin-dependent diabetes or asthma may well be manageable in children's services. It is the playroom staff and not I as director who take responsibility for the day-to-day care and education of the child. So in accepting a child with a chronic illness we must ensure that staff are completely aware and supported through this process. Any uncertainties or anxieties must be cleared up before (and after) the child commences care. We have found providing training to the whole staff team, including regular relievers, is very valuable in making staff feel more comfortable and competent when entrusted with a responsibility that they may not previously have encountered. The parents of the child concerned will also feel that your centre is a safe place, with caring and responsible staff, and that their child is well cared for at all times.

Value sharing

Young children often share their views, wishes and feelings with early childhood staff. Children's ideas and comments may be expressed in a variety of ways, through their artwork as well as conversations with staff and peers. Topics raised by children can range across many of their interests and activities, such as their favourite television programs, ambitions about jobs, who they spent the weekend with, going shopping and taking care of a pet animal. This information is rarely, if ever, systematically collated and analysed by early childhood professionals to extend their understanding of family contexts. Thus, while most early childhood professionals could identify which child has a pet animal, their knowledge and understanding about how and why families acquire pets and organise the care arrangements will be limited.

Based on research with Scottish families, Hill (1989: 195) concluded that children's experiences with their families were 'closely linked to parental beliefs and values, as well as the nature of the local neighbourhoods and network patterns'. Parents' expectations about sleeping routines, for instance, provide an opening to engage in discussing values using practical day-to-day considerations. Yet rarely do these everyday conversations go beyond the descriptive state of extracting responses to questions that begin with how, what, when or where. To extend these conversations to values-sharing opportunities requires early childhood professionals to take a proactive role, leading the conversation in directions to encourage both parties to explore the wider basis of the decision-making process at home and at the centre.

Information about children's family contexts is at times obtained and documented under crisis or difficult circumstances, such as when a parent is unexpectedly hospitalised or is required to travel overseas without taking the children. During this period, staff–parent exchanges may document possible attachment and separation issues. Through collaboration, temporary absences can be well managed by staff and parents. Documentation of potential indicators of abuse and neglect is, however, more problematical, especially as the child's comments may contradict the parents' views. Specialist training, linked to local regulatory requirements, is usually available to guide staff during these types of crisis. Emergencies and crisis situations can bring to the surface the best and the worst in individuals. Crisis situations are usually not the ideal time to engage in discussions on values. Direct questioning or asking someone to talk about their family values can also be limiting. The abstract and judgmental nature of values as well as difficulties in putting into practice one's own beliefs may get in the way of engaging in an expansive dialogue to raise awareness and promote understanding.

By critically reflecting on current practice and policy, early childhood professionals can explore their attitudes and values related to working with families. This can be undertaken as a three-stage project, as follows.

Stage 1: Self-assessment

Consider your own beliefs about working with families and document your responses in term of questions such as:

- What are my views about working with families?
- What do I consider to be the key objectives of working with families?
- What assumptions do I have about parents, families and parenting?
- What do I see as the critical differences between *my* role and the role of parents in promoting children's growth and development?
- How will I respond to families who have differing views on childhood and early education?
- How do I communicate my expectations about family involvement to parents?

It is useful to refer to the available literature on family participation in children's services, and to consider how your views are reflected in current theories and research findings. Identify any aspects from the research that you may wish to pursue further. Keep a copy of this initial assessment in your professional development portfolio and review this regularly to see how your practices evolve over time.

Stage 2: Audit of centre policies and practices

Carefully examine the ways in which families are incorporated in the ongoing activities of your centre, in program development, in centre management and governance, or in any other areas of the centre's work. Collate appropriate documentation including the centre's philosophy and policies on parent participation, and review methods adopted in maintaining communication with families. This review should include an appraisal of newsletters, notice-boards and other types of information made available to families. Consider, for instance:

- How are families involved in the day-to-day administrative matters, centre management, as well as program and policy design and evaluation?
- What mechanisms are in place to respond to complaints by parents?
- Do the centre's newsletters and noticeboards reflect family diversity?
- How does the centre evaluate its approach to family participation?

Family satisfaction with current practices can be assessed formally through a survey questionnaire or by sampling a group of families to observe and document the nature of interactions between staff and family members over a specified period of time. Some families may prefer doing a short telephone interview or an electronic questionnaire sent via e-mail to present their point of view. Family input in determining the methods of evaluation and data analysis can also engender a spirit of cooperation between parents and professionals.

Stage 3: Activate a strategic plan

On the basis of the information collected during stages 1 and 2, the extent to which there is a match between parental and professional beliefs and expectations as well as centre policy and practice can be analysed. Depending on the level of congruence achieved, new targets for working with families can be defined to redress any problems identified, as well as to test new ways of facilitating parent–staff communication. Documentation and circulation of achievements and shortcomings provide a basis for future action in a strategic way.

Continuous reflection and dialogue is necessary to sustain effective partnerships with families. The degree of involvement of families in decision-making throughout stages 1–3 also demonstrates the professionals' commitment to working collaboratively with families.

WHY DOES COLLABORATION WITH FAMILIES MATTER?

The fact remains that working with families is one of the fundamental components of an early childhood professional's everyday work (NAEYC 1993; Oberhuemer 2000). To be successful in this area, the early childhood professional needs to begin by evaluating her/his objectives and rationale for wanting to work with families. Getting to know family values and beliefs has many benefits, and there are at least four good reasons (which follow) why early childhood professionals must strengthen collaboration with families.

1. To bridge the gap between home and the service, and ensure consistency and continuity for children

Your service may be the first and only point of contact with a public institution or community service, other than a hospital or health centre, that a family has. In Western countries such as Australia, many families today live in isolation and children spend large amounts of time in child care. For instance, it has been estimated that, in Australia:

> . . . a child can spend up to 12,500 hours in child care before starting school; that's only 500 hours less than the child will spend in lessons during the whole 13 years of schooling.   (NCAC 1993: 1)

Active exchange of information between the centre and the child's family is imperative in upholding the child's sense of security and wellbeing.

2. To plan more effectively for children based on their individual needs, interests and abilities

It has long been acknowledged that parents in particular know more about their own children, yet early childhood professionals have been slow to acknowledge and access this source of information when developing programs for children placed in their care (Tinworth 1994). If early childhood professionals truly believe in making their programs more meaningful and relevant to children, they must learn to consult and listen to parents and work with them at all times rather than waiting until there is a problem (Gallinsky 1990).

3. To model cooperative social skills to children, in teaching them the real meaning of being a member of society

Early childhood services provide an ideal environment for children to experience and learn those social skills necessary for their future participation in society. We have a professional as well as a moral/community responsibility as adult members of society to pass on social skills to the next generation through demonstration or role-modelling. This view is reinforced by parents, who believe that the main reason for sending children to child care or preschool is for them to socialise with their peers (Page, Nienhuys, Kapsalakis & Morda 2001; Olmstead 1994). More attention, however, needs to be paid to how and what children observe in and learn from the interactions between parents and staff in children's services, including the importance of respect, trust and collaboration in accommodating family diversity.

4. To ensure accountability and service satisfaction to children and parents who have chosen to use your professional services

The literature on parent participation in early childhood shows that there has been a move away from being driven by a compensatory ideology to a marketplace ideology, where 'the customer is always right'. In some places this approach has moved so far that parent participation is a right enshrined in the regulatory aspects of the management of early childhood services. Some may see this as increasing the pressure and creating unnecessary tension between parents and professionals. Another way to look at it is to see the legal requirements as a way of reinforcing the importance of developing good staff–parent communication through public acknowledgment of this responsibility.

The establishment of sound and effective methods for collaborating with families is largely the early childhood professional's responsibility. Yet those early childhood professionals who believe that their main function is to promote children's growth and development through the program 'may resent and resist the idea that they must take major responsibility for establishing and maintaining the partnership' (Stonehouse 1995). How can a teacher plan for children without taking into account the child in the context of the family and society in which they are growing up? Accordingly, instead of looking at parent participation as a burden, it should be seen as an invaluable asset—

something that should be nurtured. Learning more about the family context will bring pleasure and benefits to all—the child, family and professional.

What can early childhood professionals do to initiate and maintain good staff–parent interactions? The literature is again bountiful with various strategies and methods. For example, Atkinson (1991) uses findings from a research study to discuss ways of encouraging greater participation by fathers, who are often regarded as the silent partners in child rearing. It is easier to develop a relationship with parents who are interested and willingly offer their support to services. For instance, Nilsen (1997) looks at a particular part of daily routines, separation and adjustment, and gives lots of practical strategies for collaboration. It is important to explore different avenues, as there are no fixed recipes for use in all situations, and each family and each situation can be more complicated than the one before.

Being open to suggestions and testing a variety of techniques will enhance the professional's own approach to working with families associated with early childhood services. Cross-cultural studies enable the discovery of creative solutions to common problems. To illustrate this point, consider the following excerpt by Esther Ng from Singapore, who offers some insightful perspectives on working with the families of children with disabilities.

Working with children who have special needs and their parents

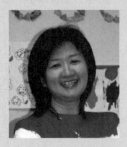

ESTHER NG
Chief Executive Officer
Harvest Centre for Research, Training and Development
Singapore

1. What does 'inclusive practice' mean to teachers and parents?

Inclusive practice has become an 'embedded practice' in my work with children and early childhood professionals. This means that it is part of my daily decision-making, on policy making for the organisation, teaching in the classroom, the hiring of employees, and working with parents. Inclusive practice requires a commonsense approach. Sometimes, it also requires innovation and quick responses to unpredictable situations. Deciding what is best for children who have additional needs takes careful thought and consideration, whether it is about the physical, the learning or the social environment.

Continued

Inclusive practice means making class rules and changing them to allow appropriate intervention to take place. It also means giving equal opportunity to every child, staff and parents to grow and learn in the same environment together, without *over*planning for the child with additional needs and neglecting others. For inclusive practice to happen in any centre or organisation, conviction has to be ignited.

2. In your experiences in Singapore, what have been some of the most valuable lessons you've learnt about working with children with disabilities and their parents?

In my early days as an early childhood caregiver, some 15 years ago, I was afraid to include disabled children because I did not know what would be best for them. During those days, my supervisor was also not interested in the idea of inclusion, I think, for the same reasons. People simply avoided the topic. So parents were turned away from centres. In the past, children with disabilities were either kept at home or sent to an institution. Today, people are more aware and more receptive to inclusion.

Sleepless nights and nightmares begin from the time parents notice that their child is quite different from other children in the neighbourhood. Their anxieties build up when it is time to register their child for primary school. Some children make it past primary 1. But soon afterwards, the anxieties build up again when parents realise that their child is not coping with school requirements and is not ready for the streaming examination at 10 years of age (that is, primary 4).

Some parents go through a stage of 'denial' and are unable to deal with the reality of their child's situation. When their children are facing learning problems in the mainstream schools, the teachers are not sufficiently trained to pick up on their needs. The common comments that come back to parents are: 'Your child is lazy', 'not paying attention', 'naughty' etc. I have found that if diagnosis and early intervention have taken place, the child can be better prepared for school. However, this does not happen in most cases. I have seen children who are diagnosed with speech, reading or even severe behavioural problems sent for assessment only when they are in primary 4—that is, when parents are at their wits' end and the final chance for a bright future in education says 'Make it through this streaming or be condemned for good'.

I am pleased that the recent proposal for the 'Remaking of Singapore' has included a very thoughtful consideration of children with disabilities. Values are caught, and not taught. In my years of working with children and families, I would often hear the cries of parents pleading for more support for their children. Today they, too, are beginning to be more vocal about their needs as parents. May their voices be heard.

3. If you had unlimited resources, what would you like to do to promote better services for children with disabilities?

Wow! If money were to drop from the sky, I would erect a purpose-built training school to support parents and teachers in the management of their children with disabilities. In Singapore, parents can go from the General Practitioner to the

Continued

> psychologist, to a speech therapist, to the Occupational Therapist and so on. Sometimes they give up for a while when nothing seems to work or they end up having to queue for a place in a special school, only to be told that it is not appropriate for their child. I hope that one day there will be a one-stop centre to go to for all disabilities, which consists of a responsible panel of qualified professionals to advise and refer these children and their families to the appropriate professional services.

It is assumed that by virtue of providing a quality service, staff will respond in a professional manner based on an accurate understanding of the centre's policies and programs. Hughes and MacNaughton (2000: 242), having reviewed the available literature on parent involvement, categorised the undervaluing of parental knowledge by early childhood professionals as inadequate, supplementary and unimportant. The extent to which early childhood professionals are able and willing to respond to parental enquiries, for instance, has not been validated comprehensively through research evidence. Nevertheless, it makes good business sense to be aware of the customers' expectations and prepared to respond cordially. The ways in which early childhood professionals define their objectives, clarify conflicting goals, ensure that all voices are heard, and find pathways to negotiate and achieve satisfactory outcomes for all, require input from children, families and professionals. As leaders, early childhood professionals can play a pivotal role in harnessing local resources, networking and bringing the community together. Oberhuemer (2000) argues that this is indeed the role transformation that is required of 21st century early childhood professionals.

EVOLVING NOTIONS OF WORKING WITH FAMILIES

Over the years, parent–staff interactions in early childhood have been variously described, researched and analysed (e.g. see reviews by Hughes & MacNaughton 2000; Rockwell, Andre & Hawley 1996). In the USA, Vandergrift and Greene (1992), who examined parent involvement in relation to children at risk, concluded that lack of success in improving parent–staff relations could be traced to inconsistencies in the way parent involvement was defined. Attempts at defining the notion of parent participation have led to the development of typologies. Scholars such as Epstein (1995) and Pugh (1996) have attempted to categorise parent participation along a continuum. The implied hierarchical nature of these typologies does not necessarily take into account societal variations arising from particular values in differing cultures.

There is much confusion about what is meant exactly when speaking about working with families in early childhood. It is unclear, for instance, when referring to parents, whether or not the term 'parents' is used in a broad sense, to include guardians and other family members (e.g. grandparents) who may have a significant role in the lives of the children using early childhood services. The early childhood literature carries a plethora of words or phrases to describe how staff and parents interact, including parent participation, involvement, consultation, representation, partners, partnerships and empowerment. Most of these terms refer to parents only, and inclusion of other family members is either implicit or ignored. Considering contemporary changes in family size and structure (such as smaller number of children per family and increasing rates of divorce) as well as lifestyle and employment patterns (e.g. immigration and high rates of work-related travel), maintaining good communication with children's families is more important than ever before.

Governments in countries such as Australia have also promoted the view that parents should be involved in decision-making in children's services (Brennan 1998a; Hughes & MacNaughton 2000; Loane 1997). Early childhood professionals, however, as Rodd (1994: 150) argues:

> ... have been slow to incorporate the full spirit of the partnership approach to working with parents because they have clung to the belief that they are the experts when it comes to children and early childhood services.

Such professionals perceived parents as lacking in parenting skills and knowledge and as requiring professional assistance to raise children successfully. Described as the 'expert model' of working with parents, the following comments capture the essence of this approach and are a timely reminder of what *not* to do:

> I who am educated and clever
> TELL YOU who are ignorant and stupid
> TO GIVE THIS TO YOUR FAMILY
> no matter how much it costs and what you usually eat
> AND THEN THEY WILL GROW AND BE HEALTHY
> and if you don't they won't grow and they will get sick and
> it will be your fault.
> (Nicholl 1985: 8, cited in Macpherson 1993: 64)

A new orientation to parent–staff relationships came about during the 1970s, which Rodd (1994: 150) describes as the era of 'communication and contact'. At that time, the focus of action for early childhood professionals was the provision of information relating to children's progress in early childhood services. During the 1980s, within an ethos of managerialism, the emphasis was on accountability to parents as consumers, and early childhood professionals were required to formalise contact with parents in relation to various aspects of service provision, including policy development and program evaluation. Yet, in assessing what happened in most Australian children's services at that time, Rodd (1994: 151) bemoaned the lack of real partnership or collaboration, describing parent involvement in service management as 'a nascent partnership'.

It was not until the 1990s that there came evidence of genuine efforts to develop partnerships between parents and early childhood professionals. For example, Ebbeck (1997) emphasised the growing belief as a result of accreditation practices across Australia that parents were the arbiters of quality in childcare services. As a result there developed a need for early childhood professionals to work with parents to enhance their mutual knowledge and understanding of child growth and development. Such knowledge can provide the foundation for high-quality child care, and assist families to identify what to look for when they interact on a daily basis with centre staff and management. However, contemporary research studies examining the net benefits of parent–staff relationships are rare and limited in scope.

Understanding the child within the context of the family is universally accepted as a primary consideration of all early childhood professionals (Ebbeck 1991; Hughes & MacNaughton 1999; Kasting 1994; Oberhuemer 2000; Rodd 1998). Indeed, it is obligatory that practitioners such as childcare staff and preschool teachers alike demonstrate their awareness and respect for working with families in their everyday practice. Yet, as Kasting (1994: 146) declares, researchers have consistently found that parent–staff relationships are 'too often strained and not meaningful'. Nevertheless, the continuity of the family as a social institution, and perhaps more importantly as a primary agent of childhood socialisation, cannot be ignored (Bronfenbrenner & Weiss 1983; Gestwicki 1992).

The current catch phrase promoting parent participation in early childhood is 'empowering families'. Langford and Weissbourd (1997: 150) describe the phrase well when they state that it represents a new kind of partnership, where the early childhood professional creates 'a welcoming environment in which parents are appreciated, not depreciated, and in which parents' confidence is enhanced, not undermined'. Empowerment is conceptually grounded within the conventional beliefs of early childhood education, where the ultimate goal is the realisation of the full potential of children during their early childhood. The new orientation, however, brings to the forefront an acknowledgment of equity in respecting the contributions being made by both parents and professionals to child growth and development.

Understanding roles and responsibilities

Authors such as Anne Stonehouse in Australia, Gillian Pugh in the UK and Ellen Gallinsky and Douglas Powell in the USA have written extensively about working with families during early childhood. These authors have commented that there is much evidence to show that working with parents is one of the most frustrating aspects of an early childhood professional's employment responsibilities. This view can be explained in part as a consequence of a lack of clarity and understanding of their roles and responsibilities as parents and as professionals. Staff responsibilities in working with parents differ according to one's employment contract, including one's status or position within the organisation. For example, as centre manager or director, the early childhood professional may have direct contact with parents when collecting fees. On the other hand, the preschool teacher's role emphasises working with families in relation to program development.

Ebbeck (1991: 178) states that parents and early childhood professionals have 'different yet mutually supportive and complementary roles', and goes on to list some of the differences between their roles (see Table 3.1).

Table 3.1 Differing roles of parents and teachers

Parents	Teachers
Parents are the most influential people in the child's early and formative years.	Teachers are highly significant people, especially when the family is small.
Parents know far more about their child than any teacher will ever know.	Teachers have a professional body of knowledge about how children grow, develop or learn.
Parents make an emotional commitment to their child.	Teachers can be objective because they see a range of children, and their teaching role is necessarily different.
Parents' commitment and contact is long-term.	Teachers are mobile, and may teach a child for a year or less.
Parents are usually not 'prepared' for parenting in a formal way.	Teachers are usually trained professionals, but in the early childhood field qualifications vary enormously.

Source: Ebbeck (1991).

Role ambiguity, where parent and early childhood professional do not have a clear understanding of what is expected of each other, is one of the primary causes of tension in developing partnerships with families. Misunderstandings arise: staff and parents view each other's positions with suspicion, and each feels undervalued by the other. Parents feel that staff have no respect for their point of view, regarding them as uncaring and irresponsible. Staff feel that parents are treating them as babysitters or servants, with little or no respect for their professional approach and expertise. Such feelings of inadequacy and/or guilt can escalate to anger and bitterness if left unchecked and unresolved.

Role confusion can also arise from people having to perform multiple roles with mixed expectations. For instance, within the context of Australian children's services, it is possible for the same parents simultaneously to adopt at least two different roles, as follows:

- ## Parents as clients or consumers

  This is the traditional view of parent participation, where the parents essentially rely on the early childhood professional's expertise and skills to enhance children's learning. Traditionally, parent contributions to program design were rare, and communication was one-directional, with the professional telling parents what was required and necessary. Over time, the nature of client/consumer and service provider roles of parents and professionals respectively has undergone significant change. Today's parents are more aware of quality matters, and as fee-paying clients they can be more demanding in seeking flexible, affordable, high-quality services which are customer-focused (Vining 1994).

- ## Parents as employers

  As Fleet and Clyde (1993: 66) state, 'getting along with the boss' is one of the most awkward and complex dimensions of parent–staff relationships in children's services. In part, this may be because the centre's owner, who is the employer, has enrolled her/his own children at the same centre and the early childhood professional has responsibility for 'taking care of the boss's son or daughter'. This situation is exacerbated when there are multiple employers. For instance, in Australia many of the non-profit, community-owned preschools and childcare centres are run by a management committee, comprising a group of about six or more parents who use the services for their own children. The centre's management committee is the legally constituted body responsible for running the centre. This means that these parents simultaneously adopt the dual roles of client and employer. With a group of parents acting as a committee, the lines of authority and communication as employers and employees may not always be clear and may increase confusion about roles and responsibilities between the parents and the professionals at that centre.

Historically, in many Western countries, including Australia, the UK and the USA, parents worked with their children's preschool teachers in a volunteer capacity in a variety of ways including helping with art and craft activities, excursions and fund-raising for the centres. However, the notion of volunteerism is also changing. Being on the management committee of a preschool, for instance, injects another layer of complexity into parent–staff relationships due to at least two factors.

First, the voluntary nature of being an employer in a preschool or childcare centre may mean that there is a knowledge imbalance. Often early childhood professionals, particularly the centre director as the employee responsible for the day-to-day centre administration, will have more expertise and be better informed, especially regarding child development and government policies, than the employer (Waniganayake, Morda & Kapsalakis 2000). The unpaid, parent volunteers, however, shoulder the legal liabilities of centre management, including determining the centre's budget and being responsible for hiring and firing staff. It is possible that some of these parents, as qualified accountants, have expert knowledge of budgets and other financial matters. Accordingly, parents and professionals bring differing skills and understanding when working together to administer and manage early childhood services.

Second, the period of parents' tenure on the committee of management is directly related to their child's need to use the service. In a preschool this may be limited to 12 months or less as is the case in Australia, because children are usually enrolled in preschool programs the year before they start school. As a consequence, there is a high turnover of committee members. This also means constant changes of employers, which can be a major source of frustration and tension for the early childhood professionals working in these services.

Without parent volunteers, non-profit services can cease to exist, as the cost of service provision is too high and cannot be contained without raising the fees. Voluntary input in centre management is also critical due to the diminishing role of government in funding and service provision (Press 1999). In Australia, community-managed, non-profit preschools and childcare centres have played a major role in establishing benchmarks for high-quality service provision. How parental, volunteer support can best be utilised is determined at the centre level. The extent of participation must not, however, be used as a criterion to assess the level of power and authority individuals have either as parents or as staff. By placing the child at the centre of interactions, early childhood leaders can reflect on better ways of garnering the skills, knowledge and resources available and accessible to everyone associated with the preschool or childcare centre.

TRAINING TO WORK WITH FAMILIES

Rodd (1998: 164) is critical that 'little specialised training has been provided for practitioners to work with adults' in everyday settings such as preschools and childcare centres, despite its centrality to professional practice and quality service provision. The persistent demand for in-service workshops and seminars on strategies to improve parent–staff communication (Waniganayake 1991) also denotes early childhood practitioners' awareness of the importance of developing and extending their skills when working with families.

Research reviewed by Epstein and Sanders (1998) shows that family participation in school-based activities varies according to a number of factors. For instance, mothers were more active than fathers overall, and the level of direct involvement declined as children moved on to secondary school. It was also clear that the onus was on the school to reach out to families and establish effective partnership practices: 'When schools select and combine activities for many types of involvement, they begin to build balanced, comprehensive and productive partnership programs' (Epstein & Sanders 1998: 393). Learning to work together to achieve objectives for the child within a school policy framework requires careful consideration. It is hard work. Staff may resist parental involvement simply as a survival mechanism, in order to remain in control and retain their status as 'experts'. Additional training input can provide guidance to bring differing perspectives together, and there is evidence to show that such action leads to stronger home–school relations.

Staff need to acquire appropriate skills to learn how to engage families and communities in children's services. The literature consistently agrees that both pre-service and in-service training can enhance staff capacity to implement innovative and effective parent–staff strategies (Foster & Loven 1992; Katz & Bauch 1999; Rodd 1998; Young & Hite 1994). In an effort to examine the interconnections of training and its impact on future practice more closely, conversations were held with three recent graduates of an Australian university who had just begun employment as preschool teachers, namely Natalie Jones, Grace Ayliffe and Merlyne Cruz. Natalie, Grace and Merlyne each graduated with a four-year bachelor's degree in Early Childhood. Their responses to three key questions are reproduced in Tables 3.2, 3.3 and 3.4 and analysed to illustrate some of the challenges of linking theory to appropriate everyday practice.

Natalie, Grace and Merlyne are enthusiastic and passionate in their approach to working with children and families. As individual early childhood professionals they found that establishing rapport with children came easily, but gaining the parents' trust was another matter. The range of challenges they each faced were similar yet different, as indicated in Table 3.2. Issues of diversity were a major concern, particularly in relation to resolving value conflicts—not only with children's parents but also with colleagues in the workplace. They were aware of the importance of ascertaining parents'

Table 3.2 What are some of the challenges that you now face when working with families?

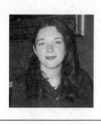	**NATALIE**	It hasn't happened yet but I am sure that the time will come when a parent's or a family's beliefs or knowledge is not in line with my own and my belief in the relevance of their knowledge will be challenged.
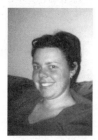	**GRACE**	Lots of issues: *non-English-speakers*, both families and children and lack of funding for translation; *confidentiality*, especially as there is very little time to chat to families without other families hanging around; *staff negativity*, which can influence my thinking and also create a vibe that shouldn't be there. Every family and every child has different concerns. It is difficult to determine when you have to agree to their demands or when you need to stick to your way of doing something. *The way that people perceive your messages*: being rushed all the time makes it hard to consider how you say things and sometimes you may sound harsher than you mean to be.
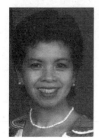	**MERLYNE**	Gaining parents' trust at the start of the year. Another challenge is convincing co-workers that we need to trust parents and to welcome their ideas as helpful insights rather than as criticisms or threats to our knowledge. Also, many parents have anxieties about their children—gender issues, behaviour management, how children cope with conflicts with other children at the centre, will they be ready for school next year, toileting etc. And parents need to know that you can handle all these issues effectively as a professional. This can be very draining at the end of the day. I am trying to discard the traditional view that teachers need to adopt an 'expert stance'.

trust early on, and accepted the difficulties they encountered in learning to manage pragmatic issues of time and energy.

Natalie and Merlyne agreed that their training did not prepare them adequately to work with families (Table 3.3). The training provided them with an appropriate theoretical orientation, but this was too narrow and limited. Grace also agreed that the training painted a rather idealistic model of parent–staff partnerships, but she found this to be helpful. She found the practicum to be restrictive in that it did not facilitate genuine engagement with families.

Table 3.3 How well did your training prepare you to handle these challenges?

Natalie

It hasn't really. For four years I trained as an early childhood professional and learnt to perceive myself as having specialised knowledge about children—all children. It was only really through my research project and the literature review that this involved that this perception was challenged: I began to think about how mainly anecdotal parent knowledge and the scientific knowledge of a university-trained teacher can both be acknowledged in work with children or indeed, whether this is possible; as I mentioned before, what happens when they clash? Whose knowledge is most relevant then?

Grace

My training definitely helped to prepare me by giving me an understanding of the ideal, and why working with families in partnership is desirable. I think that the practicums were great training grounds because, for me now, the theory tells us why, but confidence in the job is just as important. The problem with working with parents on practicums was that we were not actually supposed to advise parents: often we felt constrained so we built up relationships that were based on everything other than how the child was going. I have to now feel my way with this, and I have definitely made mistakes because I am not used to creating a whole relationship with parents.

Merlyne

At university, our conversations centred mainly on theory but not so much on practical (or real) issues such as the ones I mentioned earlier. Parent involvement has not been a major theme in my teacher training program. In my course, inclusion of family issues content was mostly limited to a number of generic subjects.

Natalie struggled to reconcile her scientific training with the parents' expectations based on informal experiences with their children. Merlyne felt that working with families needed to be allocated more time and attention in the degree program, particularly in such areas as the inclusion of children with additional needs.

The challenges that Natalie, Grace and Merlyne faced as beginning practitioners provide compelling evidence to urge early childhood teacher educators to explore alternative strategies for enhancing the use of appropriate skills when working with families of young children using early childhood services. To this end, they have offered some insightful suggestions, as indicated in Table 3.4. Natalie refers to the exploration of critical theory and Grace suggests the empowerment of students to maximise the learning opportunities available during practicum placements. Merlyne also recommends extending practical experiences to include more variety in the types of settings, beyond the traditional preschool or childcare centres to include more generic community services.

Table 3.4 If you were to rewrite early childhood training programs, what would you like to change and why?

Natalie
While the importance of parent involvement has been part of our training, I think it would be beneficial to challenge students with the concept mentioned earlier, by accepting non-scientific knowledge as just as relevant and important to our work and allowing parents' voices to really have a part in the program and the sorts of challenges that this entails. Gramsci's theory of organic intellectuals really interested me when I was writing my discussion, and that could be incorporated in training programs in line with the above.

Grace
The practicums were great because they allowed us to see how others have handled issues of working with families in real life. However, as my human services officer says, 'There are a hundred ways to do things, and it is a matter of finding the right way for you'. Certainly, there are no pat answers. I believe that you really need to have a go at understanding how theory works and be comfortable enough to practise it to find your own communication style and personality when working with families.

Merlyne
I would offer courses that addressed issues such as diverse family issues, child-rearing practices, attitudes towards families, communication techniques, conference skills, sensitivity to multicultural issues, working with families of children with disabilities/behaviour problems. I would like to see more practical, hands-on and actual training experiences with various family structures, not only through early childhood settings but through community involvement as well.

Changing conceptualisations of what constitutes a family demand that the early childhood practitioner rethinks practice, including the analysis of underlying philosophy and goals of parent–staff interactions. Assessment of teacher education programs in the USA led Katz and Bauch (1999) to declare that preparation for parent involvement was neither compulsory nor a priority in preservice training. In concluding, they reiterated the views of educators such as Foster and Loven (1992), that pre-service training must adopt a more systematic approach to fostering parent participation, and that ongoing training must be made available to practitioners working in direct services such as preschools and childcare programs.

Research consistently shows that partnerships with families are possible and necessary but require creativity, resources and mutuality in organising and sustaining them (Epstein & Sanders 1998). Natalie, Grace and Merlyne stand as effective role models of reflective practice. Their stories highlight the importance of critical evaluation being taken for granted in professional development in the early childhood field. By bringing together the views and experience of practitioners from the field with the teacher educators and the next generation of graduates from tertiary institutions, innovative solutions to the concerns expressed here can be identified, trialled and evaluated through future research.

Epstein and Sanders (1998) concluded that centre-based work needs to be placed in a broader societal context. Access to adequate resources can ensure a more comprehensive approach to partnerships, and is necessary because:

> . . . *good partnerships change teachers' attitudes about parents' helpfulness, provide parents with the information they need to remain involved in their children's education, and allow students to see that their parents care about school work and homework.   (Epstein et al., 1998: 394)*

In other words, partnerships with families have the potential to strengthen relationships across the community with those directly and indirectly involved, and the accumulated benefits go well beyond the individual child and family.

ACTIVATING PARTNERSHIPS WITH PARENTS

Studies by educators such as Emblen (1998) highlight the differing views about early education held by parents and professionals and that these differences may be linked to cultural origins. Apart from calling for greater collaboration between parents and staff, the need to engage in value sharing is rarely discussed in these studies. While the research literature on parent participation continues to grow, Young and Hite (1994) express discontent that these studies lack definition and sustained commitment to parent–professional partnerships, and that this is in part due to the complexity of the topic.

There is considerable variation between and within early childhood services regarding the types and levels of interaction between parents and staff. Some centres may view parent participation as an essential aspect of helping to contain the cost of service delivery. Rosters to undertake various tasks on a regular basis may be characteristic of those centres which are run as parent-managed cooperatives. In such centres there is a high level of input from parents, and this input may be a mandatory requirement of all families. Regular participation in helping to maintain the buildings, grounds and equipment, and attendance at various committee meetings, may be examples of how parents are expected to contribute to the centre's maintenance and management.

In other centres, such as those that are privately owned and run as a small business, parent participation is voluntary and families can decide whether or not to be involved in centre development. Parents have opportunities to con-tribute, ranging from making suggestions to change the lunch menu to helping staff set up a children's art exhibition in a shopping mall to promote the centre's work. Such options, however, usually indicate short-term, irregular commitments, and are usually tied to specific projects or events, for example open days, fundraising or excursions.

By and large, parent participation tends to be limited to conversations with staff at drop-off and pick-up times. For many parents who are studying or are employed full-time and have more than one child, taking on extra responsi-bilities to participate in the ongoing work of their child's early childhood service may be neither feasible nor practical. The onus is on early childhood professionals to find the best ways to get to know each family and negotiate the most effective means of staying in contact with them.

Usually the information that is provided in children's services enrolment records includes basic demographic details such as children's ages, parents' occupations, contact details, food allergies, and languages spoken at home. Staff need to consider innovative ways of maximising the use of this infor-mation, for instance by preparing a family profile to highlight the diversity of the centre's users. This analysis of available documentation about children's families in turn may lead to further discussions on the program or curriculum matters. The presence of a high proportion of families who speak two lan-guages can raise possibilities of introducing a bilingual program or teaching a second language at the centre. Examination of languages used within the local community is another aspect of this investigation. Families need to believe that staff are genuinely interested in getting to know them. By making use of the information that families have already provided, and which is meaningful and relevant to them, staff demonstrate enthusiasm and willing-ness to work with families. This approach enables decision-making to be both collaborative and efficient.

Rhetoric and reality of partnerships with families

Working with families is a major testing ground for professional and personal values. Both parents and professionals experience this tension from the first day they begin to share the responsibilities for a child's care and education. There is much written about the adjustments that children and parents undergo during the period of transition from home to external care (Barth & Parker 1993; Ochiltree 1994; Robins 1997; Sims & Hutchins 2001). Yet little has been written from the perspective of the professional, who is expected to know 'everything' about ensuring that transitions are peaceful and harmonious for all con-cerned. It is, in fact, taken for granted that early childhood staff are com-petent and capable professionals, who have through training acquired the necessary skills to work in partnership with families. At least that is the rhetoric of high-quality standards and the expected public behaviour. But the reality of achieving a partnership relationship with families has never been easy.

The rhetoric of partnerships permeates discussions about working with families (Ashton & Cairney 2001). The extent to which these discussions are one-sided is rarely critiqued or discussed, although much time and space is usually devoted to ensuring that the families are kept happy one way or another. The reality of the hypocrisy rarely comes to the surface because, for their part, the professionals carefully manage the process of maintaining congenial contact. Their position as 'knowledge experts' is well insulated and reinforced by the organisational structure and functions of the institutions. Parents are equally obliging, usually fearing staff reprisals against their child. This context does not augur well in nurturing the mutual trust, reciprocity and respect which are the foundations of partnerships and necessary for community building (Cox 1996; Putnam 1995).

Teamwork and shared decision making are necessary in pursuing the common goal of ensuring children's wellbeing. There is agreement that the child's 'best interests' are central to making the child feel happy, safe and secure. Yet achieving this noble goal can often feel like seeking an unreachable star. So how does one balance the scale? Is this the responsibility of the professional or the family? The commitment to pursue avenues to obtain mutual harmony, trust and respect provides solace for both professionals and parents, and therefore must be shared.

Articulating one's needs, expectations and interests as a family member or as the professional charged with the care and education of the child can seem a daunting task, and is best achieved over a period of time. It is unrealistic to think that one can find out everything and develop a full understanding of a particular child/family through a single parent–staff meeting. Parent–staff meetings, sometimes referred to as parent–staff interviews, are commonplace in most early childhood institutions. Formal meetings with individual families are an annual event, used as a reporting-back mechanism by early childhood professionals. The extent to which the parents may feel under pressure at these meetings also cannot be ignored. Not being a professional in early childhood education may result in the parents feeling disempowered, even when there are no significant concerns about their child's achievements and wellbeing. Mutual respect and empathy between parents and professionals are essential in realising partnerships.

Collaborative policy making

There is increasing acceptance that 'children's early care and education is a shared responsibility between the family and the state and not just for the family alone to bear' (OECD 2001: 40). In formulating policies that reflect a shared approach to planning, governments have to consider how to gather the necessary information to guide policy deliberations. In the following excerpt, Christine Woodrow from Australia discusses an innovative initiative established by the federal government to canvass parents' perspectives on children's services matters.

Consultation and collaboration with parents—a government initiative in Australia

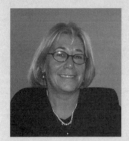

CHRISTINE WOODROW
Senior Lecturer
Faculty of Education and Creative Arts
Central Queensland University
Rockhampton

1. You were appointed as the first chairperson of the Federal Minister's Council that was set up to obtain parents' input on childcare matters. Could you please explain the reasons for establishing this council and its key functions?

The National Advisory Council on Childcare (NACC) was established by the former Federal Minister for Family Services, Senator Rosemary Crowley, to provide policy advice and advice on strategic directions in child care. I believe the establishment of the NACC, later renamed the National Parents' Childcare Council (NPCC), was a genuine attempt by our government to provide a mechanism to hear issues from the perspective of parents. At the time of the establishment of the Council, the provision of child care by the private sector was intensifying, and this was still an issue of contention in various arenas of early childhood policy. Establishment of a mechanism for 'complaints handling' was the first area that the Minister asked the Council to explore, and I think this reflected the government's concern about quality and its sensitivity to private-for-profit issues. The second major area of focus for the Council was related to flexibility in the provision of child care within the government's policy guidelines. This was a big project and an area of major concern, as both the government and Council were aware of the many inequities for parents within the existing arrangements. Shift workers, especially those working split shifts, and people employed casually were experiencing real difficulties in finding child care due to access and affordability issues. The Council spent much time and energy canvassing these kinds of issues as part of its brief.

Continued

2. How did the Council canvass the views of ordinary parents, and to what extent were these methods successful in capturing diverse community concerns?

The Council adopted a number of strategies to canvass the views of parents. These included holding meetings in places outside Canberra (the capital city of Australia), and convening community and parent forums in every state. In addition, parent surveys were undertaken, and I as president travelled widely, attending various conferences, convening forums, and visiting centres and services. The Council received letters from individuals, established a 1800 free telephone line, and promoted itself widely. I think these approaches were appropriate, and had the Council survived the subsequent change of government, there were other planned strategies to strengthen parents' input into Council deliberations. For example, a working conference specifically focused on promoting the interests and perspectives of parents had been planned. This was to be combined with an 'expo' of innovative practice, addressing the concern about lack of flexibility within services.

As president, I was developing networks and talking to people in rural and regional Australia, who had very particular constraints and challenges in accessing appropriate child care. A newsletter was to be distributed through a variety of child and family services, including childcare centres, schools and community health centres.

3. The Council ceased to exist after only two years, when the prevailing government lost the election. What were its major achievements in this time?

The establishment of the NPCC was somewhat controversial at the time, as it was the only national advisory council in the policy area of child care. Later an 'industry' council called the National Childcare Advisory Council (NCAC) was established. I still believe it is important that the perspective of parents is vigorously represented, and is not relegated to token membership on other committees. I think establishing that precedent was valuable in itself. We became a collecting point for the identification of issues of importance to parents with young children, such as childcare needs of rural farming families, care of sick children and children with disabilities using home care. In many ways the Council's agenda was overtaken by other political events, especially the federal election, which saw John Howard taking over from Paul Keating as Prime Minister of Australia in 1993. I think that the Council gained credibility as a voice for parents. Establishing forums for parent input to ensure that we had a real flavour for the issues, and meetings with various stakeholders, took much of the first year of the Council's operation.

4. Why should governments listen to the advice of committees such as these?

Committees such as these are a fundamental component of our democracy. The experience of chairing the Council taught me much about the politics of 'representation' and 'advice'. The Council was working on developing strategies to ensure that our perspectives were informed by the 'grass roots'. Most (but not all) of the Council members were active participants in the delivery of child care services, or had recent or current experiences as parent users of a childcare service. Employer groups were also represented through a member of the Business Council of Australia. I still believe that it is fundamentally important to ensure that a range of parents as stakeholders in early childhood, with differing points of view, have the opportunity to shape advice to government.

The establishment of the National Parents' Childcare Council in Australia demonstrated a commitment to open, consultative government and an evidence-based approach to collaborative policy development. There is also a growing recognition of the need to consider policies and programs for children within the broader context of the social and economic policies of a nation (OECD 2001).

At the World Summit for Children in 1990, the world's political leaders signed a declaration that read 'the well-being of children requires political action at the highest level', signalling for the first time in human history that children had become a political priority (Bellamy 2002: 3). The ambitious goals and objectives established over a decade ago in terms of child health, education and other aspects of communal living, such as access to safe drinking water and sanitation, have had some success. However, the persistence of poverty, malnutrition, inequality, armed conflict and the ravages of HIV/AIDS continues to endanger children's lives globally (Bellamy 2002).

A healthy baby with access to high-quality child care has the potential to thrive and excel at school. To achieve this requires a whole-of-government approach, where disparate departments of social welfare, health and education come together to build a comprehensive and cohesive strategic plan of action to deliver services in an integrated manner. There is also sufficient evidence to suggest that decentralisation and devolution of responsibilities to local communities has many benefits:

> Despite the inherent challenges of bringing together various services, and professionals, administrative integration has helped to promote co-ordinated and interdisciplinary ways of working, as well as a more coherent, and possibly more efficient, allocation of resources to young children and their communities.   (OECD 2001: 82)

As the front-line managers of an essential community service, early childhood professionals are ideally placed to bring together differing stakeholders to debate social policy matters from the point of view of meeting child and family needs during early childhood.

CHAPTER SUMMARY

This chapter deals with the complexities of learning to work effectively with families in children's services.

- Family diversity cuts across all aspects of service delivery in early childhood.
- In designing and implementing partnerships with families, early

childhood. professionals must begin from a basis of respecting and responding to family diversity.

- An understanding of the centrality of values in guiding interactions with families is critical to working with families.
- There is a need to examine the differing roles and responsibilities of parents and professionals.
- The necessity to continue professional training to keep abreast of current knowledge and theories on working with families was reinforced.
- In activating partnerships with families, the rhetoric and reality of current policies and programs were considered, and innovative policy developments were identified.
- Commentaries by leading early childhood practitioners in Singapore and Australia provided some insight into innovations in activating effective relationships with families.

 Discussion and reflection

1. Get a copy of a parent handbook prepared by a preschool or childcare centre. Does it include a statement about the centre's philosophy? What does this document suggest about the centre's approach to parent involvement in the centre's activities?

2. Discuss with parents in your centre/program what they mean and understand by the term 'parent participation'. Compare parents' responses with your own definition. In what ways are their views similar to or different from yours?

3. Set up a system to build a family background profile on each child in your program. As a starting point, analyse existing child records, including observations and program plans, to identify any comments or notes pertaining to the child's family background. Identify gaps in the information related to each child, and about all the children as a group, to see whether there are any overall patterns.

4. Ascertain parents' views about values education, including their expectations about the role staff should play in teaching children values. Discuss with others, especially professional colleagues, how you would handle situations where staff and parents' values are in conflict, and what needs to happen to achieve a balance.

5. Plan and run a staff development session on getting to know family values and beliefs. Topics of particular interest may include discipline, excursions, food, hygiene, sleeping routines, and vaccination. Reflect on the findings of the centre parents' values and beliefs in relation to your own beliefs and those of your local community.

6. Do you believe in establishing partnerships with families? As the professional, what will you bring to the partnership? Are there aspects or areas that you need to work on in developing better relationships with some but not all parents?

Chapter 4

Achieving quality: Cross-cultural perspectives on responding to challenges and opportunities

Quality improvement and assessment are associated with contemporary practices in most fields of employment, and early childhood services are no exception. Quality is an abstract concept, bound by culture and context. Cross-cultural perspectives of quality assurance reflect diversity in the ways early childhood professionals respond to challenges and opportunities in the provision of their services. Leaders in early childhood can explore the day-to-day issues of implementing and assessing quality in strategic and analytical ways. In seeking excellence in early childhood and with the assistance of international experts on quality issues, this chapter explores a variety of perspectives on quality assessment and improvement in early childhood services.

Outcomes

At the conclusion of this chapter, the reader should have:

- developed an understanding of quality as an abstract concept bound by culture and context;
- grasped the complexities of implementing and assessing quality;
- developed an understanding of how leaders can assist staff in implementing strategies to achieve quality;
- some knowledge of strategic ways to achieve quality outcomes.

QUALITY DISCOURSE

Woodhead (1996: 9) equated his search for a definition of quality with 'trying to find the crock of gold at the end of a rainbow. We may make progress in the right direction, but we never quite get there!'. This is an apt description, because it captures the mystery and mythology in the discourse of quality. It also reflects the confusion and lack of consensus in the definition, measurement and purpose of quality assurance in early childhood (OECD 2001). The challenge is to retain the optimism of the rainbow image, because the pressure to measure quality can undermine any potential goodness to be derived through the engagement in the search for quality.

Quality is abstract, multidimensional and difficult to measure because of 'the complex interplay of many factors' (Wangman 1995: 68). In discussing this complexity, various authors have attempted to conceptualise quality in different ways:

- Quality is a product—either as inputs or outcomes of good practice.
- Quality is a process—what is happening in programs in relation to organisational goals and objectives.
- Quality is relative—it is value-laden and culture-bound; it is also individualistic—quality is whatever the customer wants.
- Quality is transitory—it varies over time; sustainability is a major challenge.
- Quality is dynamic—perceived as a mark of distinction, quality imperatives can be highly influential in decision-making.

Above all, quality discourse is always embedded in values (Moss & Pence 1994). Values, however, are not always acknowledged or discussed; to do so requires making one's values transparent and subject to debate. When working with parents, policy planners, community groups and other professionals, early childhood professionals are ethically bound to be respectful and responsive, accommodating divergent views on all aspects of program provision to children and their families (Stonehouse 1991). This is not an easy undertaking. Values, especially personal values, can reflect deeply held beliefs and assumptions that do not necessarily sit comfortably with the professional values displayed in public.

Reviews of the research literature on quality (e.g. Ochiltree 1994) suggest that there have been three main waves of enquiry on quality in early childhood. The first wave was marked by concern about the harmful effects of child care on children's long-term development. These early studies, carried out in the 1970s, were methodologically limited, and the relevance and wider application of findings were problematical. The second wave of quality research came about in the 1980s, and looked at the diversity of child-rearing environments, including home-based care. This period saw the beginning of attempts to find objective measures of assessing quality in early childhood services. In the 1990s, during the third wave, the focus shifted to widen the debate to look at the interactive nature of quality indicators in an organisational setting, the home and the wider community context. Aspects of diversity came to the forefront during this period and remain a major challenge today as we struggle to find common understanding between the various stakeholders about what constitutes quality in early childhood.

As the 21st century progresses, it is apparent that there has also been a significant shift away from reliance on North American research to a consideration of studies done elsewhere, especially in Europe and Australia. International comparisons have reinforced the significance of the impact of a nation's cultural, historical and political forces on quality assurance in early childhood (e.g. see Hujala-Huttuunen 1996; Karrby 1999; Moss & Pence 1994; Sheridan & Schuster 2001).

Quality and culture

It is so easy to consider quality from a Western cultural perspective, as if the Western model of child rearing were universal. It is not. Neither should the Western approach to early childhood services, with their developed curricula and professionally trained staff, be the criterion on which quality services are based.

It might seem trite to say that quality is relative. It is. But the question is 'Relative to what?'. Much of the Western research on quality indicators mentions such factors as the higher child/staff ratios, the level of education of the staff, the administrator's prior experience, and the wages of the teachers and their specialised training, as being important factors in achieving quality services (Cost Quality and Outcomes Study Team 1995). If we look at the various countries around the world that have early childhood services such as child care and preschools, we cannot equate many with the economic and social levels of countries like USA, UK and Australia. It would be foolish to use the above-mentioned factors of quality appropriate to Western countries as indicators of quality, say, in Central African countries or in small island nations in the Pacific. Quality considerations can be considered only in light of the expectations and provisions of the culture under scrutiny. Indicators of quality are relative to a particular culture: they cannot, and should not, be transplanted from one culture to another. We should return our thinking to Bronfenbrenner's 'ecological systems theory' of child development to keep this matter in perspective. The multiple layers of environment surrounding the development of the child vary from culture to culture, and what is established to support this development must also be in keeping with the layers in the society of that culture. These are the complex and interacting forces, spoken of by Berk (2000), that affect child growth and development.

Responsibility for quality assurance

Quality assurance may be described as a way of supporting 'continuous improvement and striving for excellence as defined by the areas of endeavour to which the system applies' (Stonehouse 1998b: 15). The differing roles played by early childhood practitioners and parents create differing views of quality. As an example, when seeking suitable preschool programs for their children, individual parents' objectives of quality can range from looking for programs that emphasise academic enhancement to those that focus more on enhancing social interactions between children. Quality assessment can change on the basis of the presence or absence of qualified staff, the availability of resources, or which aspect(s) of the curriculum are emphasised at a particular centre. The manager of a childcare centre marketing it globally, for example, might be concerned about the centre's achievement in an international quality audit. The cook at the same centre may feel personally empowered for being awarded the highest rating by local health authorities for the food-handling strategies she uses. Accordingly, depending on their sphere of activity within organisations, quality concerns will differ between individuals. This view is reflected in Figure 4.1. As community leaders, early childhood professionals must

Figure 4.1 Quality assurance is in the eye of the beholder

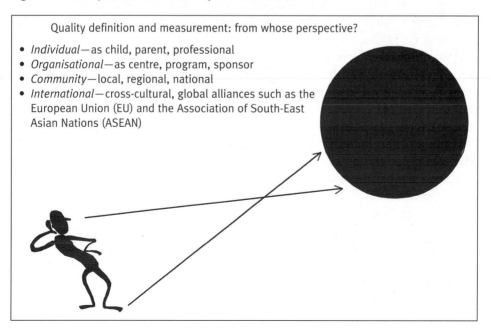

Quality definition and measurement: from whose perspective?

- *Individual*—as child, parent, professional
- *Organisational*—as centre, program, sponsor
- *Community*—local, regional, national
- *International*—cross-cultural, global alliances such as the European Union (EU) and the Association of South-East Asian Nations (ASEAN)

embrace a global perspective, taking into account internal and external drivers of quality.

In the final analysis, it is the early childhood practitioner, as a professional in her/his field of child development, who must assume responsibility for assuring that there is quality in the services she/he is providing. It may be that the owners of centres or the committees of management of centres have the ultimate responsibility for everything that happens in a centre; however, they usually delegate much of this responsibility to the professional leaders of the centre's staff. Quality assurance, as a result of such delegation, then becomes the responsibility of the professionals. This responsibility is what professionalism is all about.

By placing their thinking within global and cultural contexts, early childhood professionals can review and reflect on the complexity of quality matters against an expansive body of available literature. Widening the operational lens in this way forces the professional to access various ideas, models and methods that exist beyond the immediate local environment. As quality assessment and enhancement are global concerns and are not limited to early childhood, the opportunity to consult and analyse the views of other disciplines augurs well when aiming for excellence in any aspect of one's work. As Raban, Ure and Waniganayake (2001: 2) contend:

> . . . our understanding of the complexity of the teacher's role in young children's development will increase in sophistication only when we move outside of existing paradigms and review and reflect on our current practices.

Current knowledge and understanding about quality in early childhood services is embedded in a body of child-centred practice. High quality practice is linked to optimum child development. There is a growing body of research that supports the view that high quality children's programs, from a long-term perspective, lead to desirable outcomes for children and their families. Longitudinal research relies on studying the same setting or group of participants a number of times over an extended period of time. Although costly and difficult to sustain, such studies systematically and repeatedly track changes and can thereby clarify conflicting findings across time and settings. The selection of longitudinal studies summarised in Table 4.1 provides a taste of possibilities in relation to quality assurance outcomes for both children and their families, and full reference details in the bibliography allow direct follow-up and clarification by readers.

Quality assessment efforts can act as an investment monitor, providing a framework to evaluate a centre's achievements, including both child and staff growth and development. Governments in particular are interested in evaluating the cost-effectiveness of providing public funding to support the provision of childcare services. Early childhood professionals need to know what are the drivers of excellence in providing appropriate services for young children and their families. There is also a growing interest among

Table 4.1 Longitudinal research on quality from a global perspective

Study	Authors and location	Sample	Key findings
Effects of day care on cognitive and socio-emotional competence of 13-year-old Swedish schoolchildren	Andersson 1992 Sweden	128 children coming from eight neighbourhoods in Stockholm and Göteborg enrolled in child care before age 1 year; followed from first year of life, then at 8 and 13 years	Teachers rated the children as performing better in school subjects (particularly those who entered during the second half of their first year of life), as more creative, and as having better verbal skills
Relating quality of centre-based child care to early cognitive and language development longitudinally	Burchinal et al. 2000 USA	89 African-American infants attending community-based childcare centres; followed up at 12, 18, 24 and 36 months of age; tested for language and cognitive development gains	Higher-quality care related to higher measures of cognitive development, language development, and community skills across time
Benefits of high quality child care for low-income mothers: the Abecedarian study	Pungello et al. 2000 USA	Follow-up of the Abecedarian study on early intervention for children from low-income families. Follow-up when teen mothers were aged 21 years; 98% of the children African-American	Concluding that high-quality child care can have long-lasting benefits for teen mothers: attained post-highschool education; and had a higher average Hollingshead score than mothers of control children
Day care participation as a protective factor in the cognitive development of low-income children	Caughy et al. 1994 USA	Follow-up sample of 5- and 6-year-old children ($n = 867$) from the National Longitudinal Survey of Youth who completed the 1986 assessment	Initiation of childcare attendance before the 1st birthday associated with higher reading recognition and maths scores for children from impoverished homes

Continued

Table 4.1 *Continued*

Study	Authors and location	Sample	Key findings
Childcare quality and children's behavioural adjustment: a four-year longitudinal study	Deater-Deckard et al. 1996 USA	141 school-aged children and their employed who used full-time child care when the children were toddlers and infants; majority were European-American families	Shows few long-term negative effects of extensive use of non-parental child care in early childhood; children's behavioural adjustment (in terms of behaviour problems and social withdrawal) in middle childhood was unrelated to variations in childcare quality, but was associated with maternal stress and parenting
Day care quality, family and child characteristics and socio-emotional development	Hagekull & Bohlin 1995 USA	52 children followed from age 6 weeks to 4 years who at the age of 29 months had childcare arrangements for more than 10 hrs/week	Good quality correlated with positive expression of emotion, especially for children from disadvantaged backgrounds; boys gaining more than girls, especially in reducing fear and increasing self-competence
Children and child care: a longitudinal study of the relationship between developmental outcomes and use of non-parental care from birth to 6 years	Harrisson & Ungerer 1997 Australia	145 first-born children and their mothers were interviewed when children were aged 4 and 12 months regarding use of child care; children assessed also using strange situation procedures at 12 months	Amount and type of care had a significant impact on attachment security; use of regulated care and more than 10 hours per week was associated with secure attachment
The high/scope preschool curriculum comparison study through 23 years	Schweinhart & Weikart 1997 USA	68 children aged 3 and 4 years, of low socioeconomic status and at high risk of school failure, living in Ypsilanti, Michigan	Findings support the importance of well-defined curriculum based on child-initiated learning activities as a long-term investment strategy to create responsible adults

Adapted from Doherty-Derkowski (1995).

professionals in ascertaining whether such programs can be reproduced, especially on a large scale so that whole societies can benefit. Whole-scale duplication is, however, not appropriate, especially in terms of transplanting models derived from another country (Woodhead 1996). Instead, it is recommended that early childhood professionals review and reflect on the efficacy of a particular model against local conditions, including the availability and access to resources needed to implement the model, and the nature of political governance and stability.

REGULATING QUALITY IN EARLY CHILDHOOD

Community perceptions of quality matters also reveal differences across gender, class, cultural and age calibrations. Such differences are not surprising, given that a person's upbringing, experiences and expertise all influence lifestyle preferences as well as professional occupation. An examination of quality assessment measures used in children's services shows that it is at the community level that public and private views about quality matters are tested. Government plays a key role in funding systems of quality assurance by positioning itself as an independent and objective arbitrator on the one hand and as the protector or guardian of children's wellbeing on the other. Based on 12 countries, the findings from the OECD's (2001) thematic review show that:

> Governments promote quality improvement through: framework documents and goals-led steering; voluntary standards and accreditation; dissemination of research and information; judicious use of special funding; technical support to local management; raising the training and status of staff; encouraging self-evaluation and action-practitioner research; and establishing a system of democratic checks and balances which includes parents.   (OECD 2001: 9)

Obviously, not all of the above functions are available in a single country. Nevertheless, the OECD's review highlights the potential that governments have, as key players in quality assurance.

Eeva Hujala and Celina Kwan are two early childhood scholars who have carried out research into quality assurance in Finland and Singapore respectively. In Table 4.2 they present their views, particularly in relation to government participation in quality matters.

Table 4.2 Quality assurance: cross-cultural perspectives from Finland and Singapore

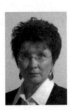 **EEVA HUJALA** Professor of Early Childhood University of Oulu, Finland	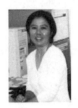 **CELINA KWAN** Assistant Professor National Institute of Education, Singapore
1. **There is an increasing interest in quality assurance in early childhood around the world. Why do you think this is and what factors are driving this debate?** I think at a macro-level this is because of social changes: more women are working, parents are better educated and want more and better services. These are the driving interests of early childhood services. Also, some or most existing early childhood services are not good enough and are causing concern among teachers, educators and professionals in early childhood. 'Not good enough' means children not being able to adjust or do well at school, especially children from disadvantaged backgrounds.	1. **Is government involvement in quality assurance in children's services essential? Why?** Absolutely, yes. Government has responsibility for *all* children. Government involvement ensures that all children have access to equal-quality child care, independently of where they live and what kind of program they are using. Government involvement therefore guarantees implementation of democracy.
2. **How should early childhood practitioners respond to demands from parents about quality assurance matters?** I think practitioners should communicate with parents, come to an understanding of what is quality and how they see quality provision. It works both ways: parents probably want to know what quality provision in all areas is, and practitioners can act as resource persons for families who depend on early childhood services.	2. **National standards on quality usually mean minimum and measurable criteria. Do you agree or disagree?** Yes and no. In addition to minimum and measurable criteria national standards must determine also the objectives for developing and improving the quality of the programs. Minimum criteria are only the foundation for quality but are not the whole quality. Quality assessment is meant to develop higher standards above the minimum regulated.
3. **You have been leading a team of early childhood colleagues to establish an accreditation system**	3. **You have been doing research in Singapore looking at quality assessment using the American Early Childhood Education Rating Scale (ECERS) developed by Harms,Clifford & Cryer (1998). What have you learnt from this research about quality assurance matters?** The ECERS areas of provision are universal and can be used in most countries. But there are areas of concern in early childhood that are unique to each nation, cultural group

Table 4.2 *Continued*

EEVA HUJALA	CELINA KWAN
for Finland. For those interested in setting up a quality assessment system in their country, what advice do you have? The first step is to train teachers to understand the importance of quality assessment for their own work. If they understand the idea and the benefits of assessment they will work hard to achieve it. All professionals must feel that they can influence the definition of quality in their own centre. Another important issue is the support teachers have from their leaders. If the administrative office supports quality assessment it will work. Quality accreditation and the whole quality improvement process must be research-based so that teachers find research-based arguments in discussions with parents, administrators and policy makers about what is professional child care and good quality for children.	or society. In Singapore, we found that three areas of academic skills— that is, reading, writing, numeracy— are missing in the ECERS. These are highly valued by parents and society here and nearly all preschools provide for these areas. I think driven by the fact that with a small market, with no natural resources, where we can rely only on human resources, these basic skills are viewed as important areas of learning. My concern is how do preschools 'teach' these skills? We attempted to include these areas into our quality research documentation, with items that described appropriate practices: developmental dimensions with lots of concrete and manipulative experiences before pen-and-paper work. I have also found that the area of bilingualism is missing from the ECERS, including the revised edition, ECERS-R. For Singapore this means teaching of three mother tongues, namely Chinese, Malay and Tamil, and this process starts at preschool. All of the research is done in consultation with local ministry officials, preschool professionals and university researchers, and this collaboration is very important in setting up quality assurance systems. Religious beliefs are another area that needs to be factored in when using the American ECERS-R in Asian societies such as Singapore.

Traditionally, governments have assumed a regulatory role in quality matters by requiring children's services to comply with the various states' licensing regulations. These regulations:

- are rules or standards which symbolise government interest and involvement in children's services;
- stipulate appropriate guidelines by dictating what are acceptable practices;
- are a prerequisite to obtaining government funding; and
- are formulated as a statutory document, not easily changed and are legislatively binding.

A licence is issued to a childcare centre or a preschool on the basis that government intervention is deemed necessary to ensure that the users of the services, especially children in this case, get a fair deal from the service providers, the owners and the staff who run the service. Regulations therefore provide legislative safeguards to ensure children's safety when they are being cared for by individuals other than their primary caregivers, their parents or guardians.

In Australia and the USA there are also multiple layers of quality assessment, including differing but compulsory state regulations and separate, additional accreditation mechanisms. In other countries such as Singapore, Finland and Japan there is a single national standard that covers child care and preschools. Gormley (1999) has effectively debated the advantages and disadvantages of government regulations in early childhood. Licensing standards tend to focus on structural aspects, such as group size, staff/child ratios and floor space. These requirements are usually prescriptive measures set at minimum compliance standards, visible and easy to measure. As a quality index, the emphasis on structural input is perceived as a weakness of regulation in that it does not get to the heart of the service being provided, namely the education and care program.

Grieshaber (2000) says that something may be regarded as regulatory if it attempts to define any direct practice of what is considered to be acceptable behaviour; behaviour that is not legitimised in this way may carry sanctions or penalties. Accordingly, licensing regulations in children's services are 'a control mechanism' (Grieshaber 2000), a way to restrain and keep in check the professionals as well as business operators who run children's services. In the long term, the net impact of this type of government regulatory system is the legitimisation and reinforcement of dominant cultural beliefs and behaviours appropriate for children during early childhood.

Accordingly, writers such as Grieshaber (2000) question the use of government regulatory mechanisms to promote quality assurance in early childhood. In supporting the need for government involvement in quality assessment, Gormley (1999: 127), however, concluded that 'at its best, such regulation can correct for market failures and offer young children much needed support at a critical time in their lives'. In the making of informed decisions as early childhood professionals, dissimilar views such as these and others that have proliferated in the literature on quality now require closer scrutiny. The following questions may be useful when comparing and contrasting different systems of children's services regulations.

What is the purpose of regulation?

The purpose is usually defined in the relevant government Acts, or in whichever legislative documents the regulations are described. The purpose of regulating may be perceived as a government's right to safeguard a vulnerable population (i.e. children). Regulation may also be prescribed as an essential role in child protection and social support, and may therefore be described as a preventive mechanism against long-term harm.

Who has the authority to enforce regulations?

Each country defines its own level of enforcement, be it national or state/local/regional governance. Enforcement and monitoring responsibilities may fall under either one or several government departments (e.g. education and welfare), a statutory board, and/or be devolved to regional or provincial authorities. Day-to-day administration at centre level may reflect tensions between the different organisational structures in terms of the level of authority each can exert on service delivery.

What is the extent of coverage stipulated in the regulations?

Considering that the types of services usually covered by regulations are preschools, childcare centres, family day care and school-age care programs, there may be different sets of standards or regulations for different types of services. Likewise, regulations may also stipulate the coverage of children's ages in different ways, such as for infants (0–1-year-olds), toddlers (2–3-year-olds) and preschoolers (4–5-year-olds). The stated divisions of children's ages within regulated children's services reflect the age of starting formal schooling in a particular country/state.

Are there aspects of regulations that will present implementation dilemmas for early childhood professionals?

The extent to which early childhood regulations are prescriptive or general varies greatly. Local administrative authorities charged with monitoring regulations can face challenges in achieving consistency and objectivity when they enforce regulations. At the same time, discretionary powers may be necessary, for instance to accommodate diversity while ensuring safety and protection for all children.

How are the licensing regulations linked to other systems of quality assurance?

Children's services regulations are issued as a licence to operate a business or service, not as an individual's licence to practise as a professional. The levels of professional training and education are usually the responsibility of authorities who are not responsible for issuing the licenses to operate early childhood services. In the matter of reaching minimum standards for buildings, equipment etc., it is important to keep in mind that the licensing of children's services must reflect related policy areas, such as building standards, health policies and fire safety requirements, that are generated by various other local authorities.

To achieve excellence in quality, are there any alternatives to regulation?

There are people who believe that, as small business enterprises, children's services are overregulated by government. Self-regulation by providers is presented as a more appropriate alternative. It could be argued that if one's objective is to achieve excellence in quality, one would be committed to delivering high quality services, for instance through the hiring of qualified early childhood professionals. Given that regulations usually stipulate minimum standards, professionals must consider achieving high quality in their services through a variety of other methods.

Other fields of study such as occupational health and safety have moved into 'performance-based' regulations. These newer regimens of quality assessment focus more on the intent of regulation, so that a higher level of output can be expected than that limited by minimum standards. One such method for working towards achieving quality services over and above minimum regulatory requirements can be through accreditation practices.

ACCREDITATION IN EARLY CHILDHOOD SERVICES

Accreditation is a relatively recent concept in Australia that is gaining the attention of governments concerned about quality assessment and improvement in early childhood services:

Accreditation is a process by which a representative body, recognised by both the service community and the community in general, establishes standards for services. These standards are above the minimum regulatory standards set by government.   (Doherty-Derkowski 1995: 113)

Accreditation has been successfully applied for some time in the health and hospitality fields as a way of promoting and marketing hospitals, hotels and restaurants. Accreditation is easily recognised by the 'star rating' systems applied: excellence in quality equates to a higher number of stars.

In the USA, the National Association for the Education of Young Children (NAEYC) established its accreditation system in 1985 as a voluntary code of practice, which childcare centres deliberately seek to secure on a fee-for-service basis. With insight gained from the NAEYC's system, some 10 years later Australia devised and launched its childcare accreditation system.

In the following excerpt, Denise Taylor, Chief Executive Officer of the National Childcare Accreditation Council (NCAC), describes her work as a leader in relation to the administration of Australia's accreditation system.

Quality assurance in children's services—the Australian way

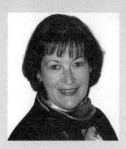

DENISE TAYLOR
Chief Executive Officer
National Childcare Accreditation Council
Australia

The National Childcare Accreditation Council (NCAC) administers quality assurance systems for children's services throughout Australia. These systems include the Quality Improvement and Accreditation System (QIAS) for long-day care centres, Family Day Care Quality Assurance (FDCQA) for family day care schemes and Outside School Hours Care Quality Assurance (OSHCQA) for outside school hours care services (to commence in 2003). These innovative quality assurance systems covering centre- and home-based child care and programs for school age children, place Australia at the forefront of international developments in quality assurance in children's services.

As Chief Executive Officer of the NCAC my key responsibilities are to ensure the consistent, equitable and timely administration of the quality assurance systems (QIAS, FDCQA and OSHCQA) throughout Australia. I manage the daily work of the NCAC, present the quality assurance systems in a variety of forums

Continued

and report to government on the achievements of the systems and the participating services.

I have spent all of my working life working with, or for children as a teacher,
an administrator and an advocate. My role at the NCAC has allowed me to move
from working with a few hundred children and teachers in a school setting to
many thousands of children and early and middle childhood educators across
Australia. The rewards of this role are many, including improvement in the quality
of programs available for children and the opportunity to work with a wide range
of people involved in the early and middle childhood professions. Working
with the quality assurance systems affirms the professionalism and dedication
of early and middle childhood staff and carers and thereby raises the profile of
these professionals. Australia is the first country in the world to have national
childcare quality assurance systems for long-day care centres, family day care
schemes and outside school hours care services that are initiated, funded and
supported by government. As such, one of my roles has been to raise the profile
of childcare services internationally through speaking at conferences and hosting
delegates from other countries.

The NCAC commenced the administration of the QIAS in 1994, and over the
first years of implementation, the progress of centres participating in the system
could be measured by the vast majority of centres maintaining or improving their
level of quality in between Accreditation Decisions. Between 1995 and 1999, over
90% of services that had progressed through the QIAS at least twice, maintained
or improved quality practices. Following a review of the QIAS, the NCAC commenced the administration of the revised QIAS on 1 January 2002. The NCAC commenced the administration of FDCQA on 1 July 2001 and will commence the
administration of OSHCQA on 1 July 2003.

Long-day care centres, family day care schemes and outside school hours care
services are each unique service types. Thus, while the QIAS, FDCQA and
OSHCQA are similar in terms of the process, there are some distinct differences
between the systems that take into account aspects unique to each service type.
For example, the quality practice standards are specific to each type of care and
the 'Validation Visits' conducted by trained NCAC validators are arranged to
accommodate the settings unique to the service type. Family day care is delivered in multiple settings, thus validators visit both the scheme and a selection
of carers, whereas long-day care is delivered in a single setting and the validator visits the centre only. Final decisions about the procedures for validation of
outside school hours care services will be made following field testing and
consultation.

The fact that the Australian federal government has funded and supported
these quality assurance systems has brought a number of benefits to the childcare field. First, community awareness of the work and value of the early childhood profession has been raised. Second, many resources for children's services
are now much more accessible on a national basis due to wider networking and
sharing of ideas among professionals and services across States and Territories.
This has also resulted in a national exchange of ideas relating to good practice,
which means that childcare services across Australia can benefit from the experience of other services. Finally, agencies outside the early childhood field are
now targeting childcare services and adapting their resources, kits, information
and so on to the needs of children's services. This is particularly evident in the

Continued

health and safety area where a number of resources are now produced specifically targeting childcare services. The NCAC anticipates similar benefits for the middle childhood field following the implementation of OSHCQA.

As an educator and advocate for children, I am proud of Australia's quality assurance systems and their impact on quality standards in children's services throughout Australia.

In both the Australian and USA systems of accreditation, the processes of self-assessment and collaboration with colleagues are central to the realisation of accreditation status (Bredekamp 1999; Duff, Brown & Van Scoy 1995; Murray 1996). Herr, Johnson and Zimmerman's study of over 100 accredited centres in the USA showed that 'overall the self study was rated as even more beneficial than the on-site validation visit' (1993: 4). In contrast, Murray (1996: 13), looking at the Australian system, issued a warning that we must not rely solely on self-ratings, and that supplementary data must be collected from a variety of stakeholders (including parents and children) and from a range of evaluative methods. Although direct input from children is not included in the Australian quality assurance system, a variety of strategies are deployed in determining accreditation status. More information is available at the NCAC's website (http://www.ncac.gov.au).

TOOLS OF QUALITY ASSESSMENT

Gormley (1997: 32) captures the essence of the quality debate by stating that 'child care is a labour problem, an administrative problem, a regulatory problem, and of course a familial problem'. In selecting the type of measuring instrument(s) that best meets one's objectives for quality assessment, one needs to be clear about who is going to do the assessment, and for what purpose. According to Scarr, Eisenberg and Deater-Deckard (1994: 132), there are three basic aims of quality assessment. Is it for the purposes of:

1. **Regulation?** Governments define the ground rules for consumer satisfaction for those using children's services. Licensing standards ensure child safety and wellbeing at a minimum level.
2. **Program improvement?** Program improvement is of interest to both consumers (consisting of the children and their families) and the service providers (including staff and service sponsors). Managing program quality therefore may be perceived as a joint parent–staff responsibility.
3. **Research?** Scholars have explored the effects of variations in quality child care over time and across differing variables in order to evaluate outcomes for children.

In effect, the type of tools utilised will depend on the users' specific interests—be these users governments, consumers, early childhood professionals or researchers—as well as the goals and objectives they have for engaging in quality assessment. For the purposes of regulation, one cannot go past existing basic regulatory regimens as discussed earlier. In relation to the quality of programs, both input and process indicators of quality (see Table 4.3) and their interrelatedness must be considered. From a research perspective, it has been shown that 'a short, simple scale is acceptable to assess process quality in child care centres in settings with great variability in quality'. This is good news because research on outcomes of quality, for instance, can be done in 'much more efficient and less costly manner than previously thought' (Scarr, Eisenberg & Deater-Deckard 1994: 149).

When undertaking quality assessment in early childhood, one must also consider the indicators against which one will measure and adjudicate the level of quality achieved. Woodhead (1996: 38) states that quality indicators are usually grouped under three broad categories, consisting of input, process, and outcome indicators. These indicators have been reproduced with minor changes in Table 4.3.

Table 4.3 Quality indicators

INPUT indicators: easy to define and measure	PROCESS indicators: reflect relationships and day-to-day interactions	OUTCOME indicators: reflect the impact of using services
• **Building and grounds** (e.g. floor space, toilets heating/cooling) • **Materials and equipment** (e.g. toys, furniture, teaching resources) • **Staff** (e.g. qualifications, wages and conditions; child/staff ratios)	• **Style of care** (e.g. adult's responsiveness, consistency) • **Teaching/learning methods** (e.g. cater to individual needs control/support) • **Experiences offered** (e.g. choices, variety, routines and transitions) • **Control and discipline** (e.g. boundaries, rules, management) • **Relationships among adults** (e.g. respect, trust) • **Relationships between staff, parents and others** (e.g. open, welcoming, cooperative)	• **Children's health** (e.g. growth levels, illness) • **Abilities** (e.g. overall skills and development) • **Adjustment to school** (e.g. transition and achievements at school) • **Family attitudes** (e.g. parent competence and support for children's learning at home)

Adapted from Woodhead (1996: 38).

By using these indices in differing ways, specific instruments (such as early childhood checklists and environment rating scales) and national systems of quality accreditation (such as the QIAS in Australia previously discussed) have been developed. One of the best-known rating scales, developed by American researchers Harms and Clifford (1980), has been 'tested' widely on an international scale in countries such as Australia, Singapore, Portugal and the UK. The Early Childhood Education Rating Scale (or ECERS, as it is popularly known) consists of 37 items categorised under seven dimensions, covering a mix of input and process indicators identified in Table 4.2. There are advantages as well as risks in the universal application of rating scales such as these (OCED 2001: 68). Kwan, who used the ECERS in Singapore, identifies some of these challenges in Table 4.2.

Concerned about the universal application of dominant Euro-American models of quality, Woodhead offers the Practice Appropriate to the Context of Early Development (PACED) framework as an alternative:

> It identifies a process of contextual appraisal of the appropriateness (hence quality) of child care environments, practices and approaches to learning and teaching. It builds on knowledge of the universal features of children's development as well as on contextual variations; it articulates how these reflect both invariant maturational characteristics of the human infant as well as variables and changing developmental niches.   (Woodhead 1996: 69)

The essential strength of the PACED framework is that it enables diversity to flourish while assessing quality in respectful and meaningful ways. Taking into account local concern and possibilities for quality assessment in early childhood, a team led by Oulu University researchers developed an innovative quality assessment framework in Finland. In the following excerpt, Eeva Hujala and Sanna Parrila present a general overview of this system.

Developing an early childhood quality evaluation system in Finland

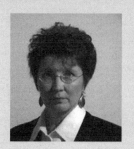 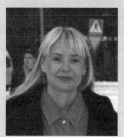

EEVA HUJALA AND SANNA PARRILA
University of Oulu
Finland

In Finland, the 'Quality Strategy' for the Public Services (1998) emphasises that economically produced, good-quality services are the central platform of the nation's ability to remain competitive in the global market. To this end, the

Continued

customer has an advance possibility and a right to know what kind of service s/he can expect. This is how citizens' rights as stakeholders and customers of public services, and as evaluators of their functionality, are realised.

The project on Quality Evaluation in Early Childhood Programs was conducted between four universities, twenty two municipalities, four provincial offices, the National Research and Development Centre for Welfare and Health (Stakes) and the Association of Finnish Local Authorities. Accordingly, it brought together early childhood practitioners with those such as researchers, trainers, trade unionists and provincial officials in the planning and implementation of the project.

Based on theory and research in early childhood, 19 quality indicators were identified. For each quality indicator, specific objectives and requirements linked to local legislation were identified. The quality requirements are fundamentals of practice that can be evaluated at the level of action. Linked to state legislation, the requirements define minimum standards and are binding. This work led to the generation of a quality management document, prepared by participating centres. The reports subsequently obtained collectively provided an evaluative base for quality review and development work at the provincial level. Close cooperation within the whole early childhood community, including parents and children, was essential in the specification of the criteria and evaluation of their realisation.

The conceptual model of quality evaluation developed through this project is illustrated in Figure 4.2. It reflects the interaction and interdependence of the contextual and structural forces of day care. In effect, its success was dependent on cooperation between the various layers of participants' contributions to quality.

Figure 4.2 Quality evaluation model of day care in Finland.

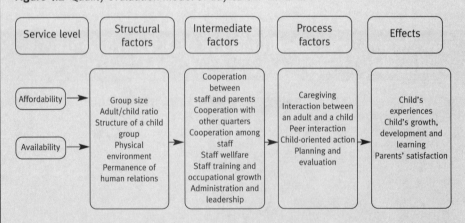

During the development phases of the project, for instance, municipal and individual practitioners were supported through local networks and long-term quality-related in-service training provided by the University of Oulu. One person responsible for day care quality from each municipality participated in this train-

Continued

ing, returning home to transfer acquired quality knowledge to others in his/her municipality.

The project team emphasised municipal responsibility in the development and realisation of quality management. It recommended the formation of municipal management teams or the appointment of a coordinator of day care within the provinces to supervise and support quality management and development of children's services.

In this Finnish model of quality assurance, input and process indicators are aligned with child outcomes. One of its main strengths is the 'participatory approach' (OECD 2001), made explicit in all aspects of the design, implementation and evaluation of the system. This model, therefore, not only makes it possible to find out 'how the children are developing' but enables practitioners to explore their practices, 'leading them to constructive self assessment and change' (OECD 2001: 71).

Administering and managing quality assurance—a generic model

One of the main tasks of an early childhood leader is to coordinate the procedures leading to quality assurance, including observation, documentation, reflection and action. Reflecting on the American system, Bredekamp (1999: 60), for instance, concluded that 'in our experience, the administrator's knowledge and skill is the most important predictor of success in a program becoming accredited'. Taking into account various stages of administration and management of quality assurance, a generic model consisting of four core functions is presented in Figure 4.3. Within this generic model, the four core functions of quality assurance consist of:

- self-assessment,
- external validation,
- certification/endorsement, and
- enrichment.

These functions are interrelated and interdependent. The way in which connections between the four procedures are established depends on how the model is implemented in a particular context. For example, by collating the self-assessment reports of a group of staff in one setting, one could identify the group's professional development needs. This information may be used to arrange for an external specialist to visit the centre to deliver an on-site consultation or in-service training session for all staff. Such enrichment activities do not have to be held back until external validation and endorsement functions are implemented, and can be provided at a time determined by centre staff and/or management.

Figure 4.3 A generic model for quality assurance.

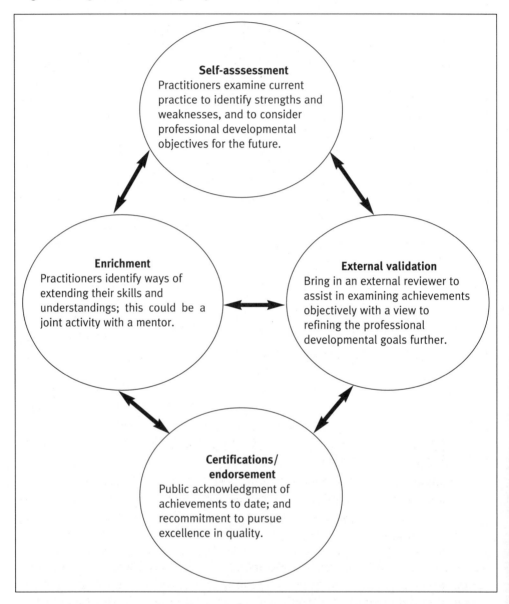

Input from other sources may be obtained in the form of external expertise or collegial support from within an organisation, including feedback from other staff as well as parents and management. To this extent, quality assurance should be perceived as a joint venture or method of collaborative learning. Public endorsement is also desirable as a way of gaining closure and demarcation between one stage of quality improvement and the next. Systematic documentation serves as a benchmark against which improvements of quality can be reviewed.

Conceptualised as a journey, this cooperative approach to quality assurance requires forward movement, where the practitioner continues to define goals and objectives for continual renewal of professional growth. The processes of learning can be enhanced through mentoring at different stages of the journey. It is suggested that practitioners develop and maintain a portfolio of evidence that illustrates the journey as it evolves. Such evidence should consist of a mix of information, that which can be shared with others as well as that which is personal—to be disclosed only at the discretion of the individual practitioner. Individual career goals, mistakes and achievements can carry deep personal meaning, and privacy is essential to building trust in the organisational context. As Woodhead (1996: 42) says:

> ... defining quality in an early childhood programme is not a once-and-for-all process. Negotiation and renegotiation are continuous. An important feature of this process is that stakeholders become more aware of their own (and others') partiality, more aware of the personal, cultural, institutional and hierarchical con-straints on the perspectives adopted, and thereby more open to the possibility of change.

The notion of a generic model describing core functions of quality assurance in early childhood implies the existence of a streamlined system that follows a linear path either explicitly or implicitly. There is the danger of reduction-ism, whereby the peeling back of the system to its bare bones (i.e. four core functions) undermines the complexity of any early childhood service. It ignores the dynamic and transitory nature of quality assessment, where changes to any single component can affect the entire system. For example, when training and education are used as an intervention without systemati-cally addressing other aspects of quality, 'the gains may not be maintained' (Buell & Cassidy 2001: 211).

It is suggested that the generic model described here be used as a starting point, equivalent to the building blocks of an accreditation system. To achieve sustainable quality, a comprehensive approach to assessment, evaluation and enrichment must be adopted. Local conditions need to be incorporated in a comprehensive accreditation package that reflects a holistic system of quality assurance. Of course the challenge remains, as Bredekamp (1999: 59) contends: 'when accreditation relies on rating scales and checklists, as it must, it is very difficult to communicate that the whole is greater than the sum of its parts'.

QUALITY ASSURANCE—KEYS TO PROFESSIONAL GROWTH

Quality assurance can enhance overall workplace practices by nurturing the professional growth and development of practitioners. Research has consis-tently shown strong correlations between quality care and aspects such as staff/child ratios (Howes 1983; Howes & Rubenstein 1985), staff training

(Clarke-Stewart 1987; Kontos & Stremmel 1988), and staff job satisfaction and turnover (Phillips, Howes & Whitebrook 1991; Phillips 1987; Whitebrook, Howes & Phillips 1989; Whitebrook 1996): 'Consensus is building regarding the importance of professional preparation and training of those who care for and educate young children' (Duff, Brown & Van Scoy 1995: 81). More recent studies have specifically highlighted the importance of compensation or wages 'in discriminating among poor, mediocre, and good quality child care centres' (Buell & Cassidy 2001: 210).

The roles of the various staff in early childhood centres in relation to quality assurance must, however, be considered beyond the basic structural considerations of qualifications and staff/child ratios. The nature of staffing, from a governance perspective as well as from an interactive perspective, must take into account staff dispositions, skills and ethics. Staff contribution to a centre's overall productivity can be assessed by exploring the achievements of individual staff. The long-term benefits of rewarding staff for their commitment and dedication are rarely discussed in quality discourse. Employer-supported professional development nevertheless can go a long way towards raising morale and standards of professionalism. When professional development is systematically built into the centre's evaluation processes it can lead to rich dividends all round.

Discussing the historical roots of quality assurance schemes in the UK, Fish (1991: 23) proclaims: 'the problem, of course, is that though the vocabulary used can be made to sound the same, producing teachers is not at all like producing arms and electricity'. This product-based, industrial approach to quality assurance is geared towards achieving customer satisfaction 'as cheaply as possible with the end product, the standards of which were clearly defined beforehand' (Fish 1991: 24). Use of performance indicators is a more recent evolution of the industry/business genre of quality assurance systems. It is assumed that performance indicators that are easily observable and measurable provide structure and objectivity. Described as a technical-rational model of quality assurance (Fish 1991), it ignores such human qualities as beliefs, values and attitudes as well as the consideration of ethics of practice.

Learnings acquired through cross-cultural research demand that we remember that 'the same practices may have different significance in the interpretation of quality criteria depending on goals, values and cultural conditions' (Karrby 1999: 22). The promotion of critical reflection as best practice in recent times offers new possibilities for future professional growth in early childhood. As Jones (1995, cited in Carter & Curtis 1998: 209) states:

> ... *professionalism is defined by reflection on practice. To reflect, we must tell our stories and give names to our experience, names that connect it with the values we hold and the theories that inform our work.*

Accordingly, early childhood professionals can engage in quality assessment on an individual basis by beginning with an exploration of their own beliefs, practices and experiences. A starting point might be when a practitioner begins to question his/her current practices relating to ongoing challenges faced in meeting the needs and interests of a particular child. The relationship between professional growth and quality matters is not always made explicit in the research literature. That is, while the link between training and quality is well established, how to use the knowledge and documentation generated through accreditation procedures, for instance, is not discussed adequately.

Self-assessment measures are generally supported in the quality literature (Al-Otaibi 1997; Eisenberg & Rafanello 1998), and are incorporated in existing systems of accreditation in Australia (Wangman 1995). Concern expressed about self-assessment by early childhood professionals covers the inherent bias associated with the subjective nature of reporting and documentation (Kelly 1992), and the higher workload, usually unpaid (Lyons 1997). Self-evaluation is nevertheless generally regarded as a 'user-friendly' way to start quality improvement. Its flexibility and adaptability in responding to individual needs, interests and abilities is strengthened by its ability to provide a meaningful reference point, a baseline against which professional growth and progress can be measured. In other words:

> . . . just as self-initiated activity is critical to the child's development, so are reflection, self-evaluation, and self-direction critical to the process of professional development.   (Duff, Brown & Van Scoy 1995: 83)

POLITICS OF QUALITY ASSURANCE

Discussions about quality assurance in early childhood are inextricably tied up with relationships of power. Social interactions based on the exercise of power may be described as politics: 'it is about determining who gets, what, when and how' (Thio 1994: 304). The arena used for political activity varies over time, and is not limited by the organisational structure (e.g. a childcare centre) or number of stakeholders (e.g. parents, professionals and politicians) involved. Inevitably, questions about quality assurance revolve around three competing forces (see Figure 4.4), concerned with:

1. authority in decision-making,
2. costs of implementing the system, and
3. definitions and measurements of standards used to assess quality.

It is possible that these three forces, either singularly or jointly, undermine the purpose of quality assurance. Conflicting or opposing purposes can create

Figure 4.4 The politics of quality.

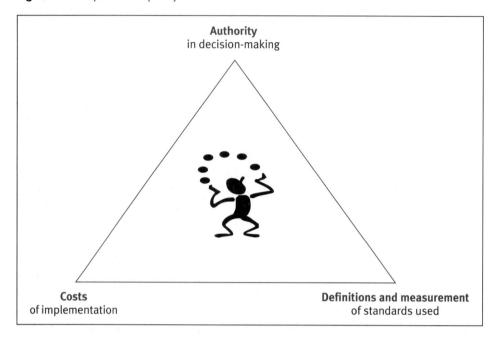

Authority
in decision-making

Costs
of implementation

Definitions and measurement
of standards used

confusion and havoc due to dilemmas arising through differing views being presented by various stakeholders.

Collaborative action between the stakeholders can not only enhance day-to-day communication but can also act as a catalyst to initiate change. Joint activity allows the different players to observe and appreciate the contributions being made by others. Knowledge of each other's roles and responsibilities can also help to consolidate relationships and thereby make the process of quality assurance more holistic. The way in which this influences decision making on quality assurance will depend on the use of power and authority vested in each of the stakeholders.

The adoption of a comprehensive approach to quality assurance relies on the use of a mixture of qualitative and quantitative tools as well as consultation with all stakeholders, especially children. According to Barclay and Benelli (1996: 91), input from children is of particular importance because as the direct recipients of services they are 'in a unique position to judge the quality of their early childhood programs, and hence can be an important source of information'.

Increasingly, emphasis is being placed on acknowledging and incorporating children's perspectives in quality matters, and this shift in attitude is closely aligned with:

> ... two complementary principles ... A belief in children's rights (including the right to be heard, to participate, to have control over their lives) and a belief in children's competence (to understand, to reflect, and to give accurate and appro-

priate responses). Together these beliefs imply that it is both ethical and logical to ask children what they think.   (Brooker 2001: 163)

In Denmark, for example, children must be included in the planning and implementation of daycare programs, as this is perceived as one way in which early childhood professionals may demonstrate their respect and regard for children's opinions (Langsted 1994: 30). Before implementing any changes to existing systems of quality assurance, it is also wise to start the process correctly. In Denmark, for instance, they started by actually taking time to observe and listen to children as citizens in their own right. In doing so they audited current practices—(this is always a good starting point because it provides a baseline against which changes can be evaluated). In order to attest to the influence that children's voices have exerted on decision-making debates, wider applications across multiple settings over a sustained period are required.

One argument put forward by critics of government intervention emphasises the need to consider the perspectives of the divergent stakeholders. Grieshaber (2000) declares that Australia's childcare accreditation system, for instance, has been deliberately couched in an outcomes-based framework; is aligned with an economic rationalist philosophy; is logical and efficient; and provides an excellent tool for public accountability. This approach is directly in contrast to the traditional approach to the non-compulsory early years of education, which was based on professional autonomy and commitment to ethical practice. From an inclusive perspective, Grieshaber (2000: 3) argues that government policy systems such as childcare accreditation can very subtly undermine diversity by ignoring minority perceptions.

Assessment, evaluation and measurement are three key terms usually linked to quality assurance. The meaning of each term and the way each is applied in practice can vary significantly among early childhood professionals. For instance, Jalongo and Mutuku (1999: 126) state that while teachers may talk of assessment in relation to individual children's achievements, 'administrators tend to think in terms of evaluation at the programmatic or policy levels', and such variation makes it 'difficult to arrive at a meeting of the minds'. Factors such as belief systems within the organisational context, stakeholder power and influence especially in relation to decision making, and responsibility for adjudication and implementation of recommendations, can all act as impediments to quality assurance. To counteract the tendency to make a program look better or more needy than it is, 'the current trend is to develop inter-disciplinary and inter-agency evaluation teams so that no one person bears all the responsibility' (Rockwell & Buck 1995, cited in Jalongo & Mutuku 1999: 131).

The use of audit teams for quality assessment is common within higher education, for example, and there is much controversy about the actual benefits of this practice (Bell & Harrison 1998). As in the case of childcare centre accreditation, external audits require the collation and completion of vast amounts of documentation as 'evidence' of quality practices. No-one enjoys this sort of paperwork, and there is never any direct financial reward for doing it. External validation by peers, however, can be satisfying in extending one's knowledge base by making one more aware of alternatives as practised in other like-minded institutions. Peer mentoring also occurs, as a part of the consultative processes of data collection and review. In fact, the training that is provided as a part of becoming an auditor or validator is recognised as invaluable professional development:

> There is now a growing body of evidence to indicate that assessors are able to take back to their own institutions examples of alternative, and often better ways of planning and delivering curricula.   (Bell & Harrison 1998: 143)

Inevitably, discussions about quality are tied up with politics, at the centre level or within the profession or the community at large. Everyone has a view about quality. As Bryce (cited in Loane 1997: 119) declares, 'quality can be intangible, a gut feeling, the sense and spirit of a place as you walk through the front door'. It is therefore highly desirable that divergent perceptions of quality be considered when identifying objectives to evaluate children's programs.

It is of course possible and plausible that personal objectives about quality will not necessarily match those of the organisation or the collective, whether it is the centre's management or group of staff in a particular team or centre. A clear statement of objectives can make the processes of quality assurance more transparent and easier to administer and analyse. Be aware, however, that finding consensus within a collective is problematical and may not even be a realistic proposition in some instances. Opportunities to engage in discussion and debate are nevertheless essential if common ground is to be found. As a leader, the early childhood professional's role is to engage the stakeholders in continuous dialogue, networking and genuine collaboration. In seeking a middle path, Woodhead (1996: 10) declares that 'quality is relative but not arbitrary'. Continuing his metaphor of quality as a rainbow, he says:

> ... as with a rainbow, we may be able to identify invariant ingredients in the spectrum of early childhood quality, but the spectrum itself is not fixed, but emerges from a combination of particular circumstances, viewed from particular perspectives.   (Woodhead 1996: 10)

CHAPTER SUMMARY

This chapter has attempted to present quality as an abstract concept bound by culture and context.

- Quality improvement and assessment are contemporary practices in early childhood services.
- Issues surrounding the regulation and achievement of quality outcomes are very complex.
- The role of the leader is crucial in helping services in their quest for quality assurance and quality outcomes.
- Issues surrounding regulation and accreditation were examined.
- Some discussion on national and international cross-cultural perspectives on quality was presented.

Discussion and reflection

1. Debate: should quality assurance in children's services be voluntary or mandatory?

2. How can we involve children in quality assurance? What strategies can you use, and why?

3. Considering the existence of parallel quality assurance systems in countries such as Australia, what are the benefits of having more than one system within a single country?

4. With increasing demand for public accountability, has quality assurance in early childhood become politicised? Who has the power to define what counts as quality in your organisation?

5. Can quality assessment be influenced by one's cultural and theoretical orientations? If so, what are the implications for external validation during an accreditation visit?

6. Discuss with your family and/or work colleagues your beliefs about what constitutes quality. Are you able to identify more similarities or more differences in perceptions of quality amongst those you consulted?

Chapter 5

Pathways to policy: Influencing and achieving positive outcomes

This chapter is concerned with how public policies are created, developed and implemented through sound administration, management and leadership. It also examines the crucial role that management policies play in the effective operation of early childhood services and the early years of school.

Outcomes

At the conclusion of this chapter, the reader should have:

- developed an understanding of the theoretical bases of public policy making;

- grasped the concept of policy making at the early childhood services level, both macro and micro;

- a better understanding of how early childhood staff can influence public policy;

- more understanding of the ways of working with staff and committees to develop policies for administration, management and leadership in services.

Effective policy making is vital to early childhood services, although to staff it can sometimes seem unrelated to the grassroots functioning of a service. However, without an understanding of the effects of policies, services can find themselves in the precarious position of closure or near-closure. As Farmer proposed (1995: 3): 'Policies are meant to spell out how your service puts its philosophy and goals into everyday practice and may affect families, community, children, management and staff'.

In 1997, the Australian Early Childhood Association (AECA) wrote:

> *In the face of falling enrolments, changes in Government policies and economic pressures, all centres need to examine their current practices and decide where changes can be made so that the twin goals of providing quality care and being financially viable are achieved.   (1997: 5)*

This indicates how seriously a professional association took government policies, including economic ones affecting the viability of early childhood centres in the face of funding changes.

Likewise, in the US early childhood publication *Young Children*, an article entitled 'Public Policy Report' (1996) stated that public officials should be held accountable for making decisions that affect children's wellbeing and learning. Supporting families in policies that invest in children is seen to reap the greatest long-term rewards. In a publication in *Rattler* (2001: 15), it was stated that:

> *A number of difficulties may arise if there are no written policies. These include decision-making problems—inconsistent and uninformed decision-making based on opinions, biases or wishes, decisions may be made that exclude relevant people, management or staff may make decisions in response to specific problems as they arise. This can lead to different decisions being made for similar situations; and confusion and conflict can arise between staff, families and management.*

Writing of policy concerns in the OECD Thematic Review of Early Childhood Education and Care Policy, Hayes and Press (2000: 28) stated:

> *There are a number of current policy concerns facing the provision of Early Childhood Education and Care (ECEC) in Australia. These include the appropriateness and effectiveness of quality assurance, the impact of a range of developments in the field on the capacity of ECEC settings to improve or maintain levels of quality, and the number of children who do not currently benefit from investment in ECEC.*

Other policy concerns were noted in the OECD thematic review, but suffice it to say that current policies in early childhood education and care relating to a range of issues did not come up to scrutiny, and even now remain as areas of concern.

It is therefore vital that early childhood staff understand the process of public policy making and its influence at national and local levels. Here it is necessary to look at public policy and the role that governments play in shaping it. A vital question emerges.

WHAT IS PUBLIC POLICY?

Public policy can be defined as the authorised rules and regulations by which organisations and bureaucracies function. Policies, in effect, establish the parameters that guide coherent decision making by personnel in organisations, however these are defined.

Policy is concerned with seeking to make organised activity stable, predictable and accountable. Razik and Swanson (2001: 257) write that 'any organisation, government, business, industry, voluntary or charitable association needs to agree on a set of rules under which it will operate'. These rules are sometimes called policies, and regulations are generated under these policies. Viewing this practice in government terms, it is about decisions made by government to undertake specified courses of action.

Public policy in essence refers to the public sector—that is, organisations and bureaucracies that deal with matters influencing and/or affecting the nation, state or, closer to home, the community. In Australia, for example, there are federal, state and local governments, all of which make policies in accordance with stated, overarching government policies. Public policies are perceived by the community as a statement of direction, intention, position, beliefs and values.

Policy then is a way of shaping actions, and without clear directions all forms of organisations are likely to become dysfunctional or at least unclear about agreed procedures and courses of actions.

Fenna (1998) writes that there is virtually no area of life in which modern government is not concerned; therefore, public policy covers a broad range of issues, which often affect one another.

Bridgman and Davis (1998: 8) propose that policy is the means that governments use to pursue their objectives. To this end, a statement of public policy is in the Australian system a statement of political priorities. Policy then becomes an expression of the political will of a government. However, Fenna (1998) draws our attention to the fact that there is sometimes a gap between word and deed. There is a difference between what governments state they are doing in their policies and what is actually happening. In explaining this apparent dichotomy, Colebatch (1998: 37) says that policy has both a vertical and a horizontal dimension. The horizontal dimension is what government policies state should happen. The vertical dimension is what happens in practice. Policy has to be much more than mere rhetoric, and there must be a clear intention on the part of the policy maker to make it work.

Bridgman and Davis (1998: 12) note that 'a government stands or falls on its policy choices. It must ensure sufficient coordination so that one policy does not undermine another'. They also endorse Fenna's point, that policies mean nothing without the capacity to implement government decisions. There is, therefore, a challenge to any government to negotiate sound and appropriate policies which complement rather than undermine other policies and which can be resourced so that they can be implemented.

THE CONTEXT FOR PUBLIC POLICY DEVELOPMENT

All public policies are situated in government and at all levels of government. In the Australian context governments gain their authority through an established electoral system. Government makes laws, has an executive comprising government ministers, administrative agencies, statutory authorities and judicial courts, all of which interpret and apply the law. Bridgman and Davis (1998: 10) cite from 'The Republic Advisory Committee' as follows:

> The Australian form of Government draws on Australian colonial traditions, British concepts of responsible government and American models of federalism. The result is a written constitution . . . the major features of which are a federal division of power, a strong parliament, a separate Australian judiciary which reviews the constitution, the validity of legislation, and an Australian representative of the monarchy who exercises nearly all his or her functions on the advice of the executive and who performs the national ceremonial role normally associated with a head of state.

In Australian parliaments there is what is called a Cabinet, which is a meeting of the various government ministers and is chaired by the Prime Minister (or, in state governments, by the Premier). It is in Cabinet that the Prime Minister (or Premier) sets the political agenda. An effective Cabinet that works in close concert with the Prime Minister (Premier) is essential for sound policy development. Cabinet membership is not static and will change over time as ministerial portfolios are altered or regrouped. The Prime Minister (Premier) decides on the size and membership of Cabinet. Although Cabinet has no legal standing within the Australian Constitution, in practice it performs many important functions, and the formulation of public policy is one of its key roles. In summary, the functions of Cabinet are:

- to act as an information-gathering and clearing house;
- to share information across the diverse range of political portfolios;
- to act as a coordinating body whereby consensus can be achieved in the face of competing demands by different ministries. Unification of purpose can be achieved within the broader government spectrum;

- to set targets and strategies for policy implementation; and
- to make policy decisions within existing laws.

It has been stated that the ministers are the executive arm of government, and they take responsibility for policy directions of government. They are accountable to Parliament for the monitoring and implementation of government laws and policies. Ministers are assisted by departmental staff, political advisers and consultants, who work in and for governments implementing policies. Therefore, policy advice and the administration of it are closely integrated in the work of government.

The model described here of government policy development has some similarity to other democratic societies. The important factor is that government, whatever the structure of the country, is the body that creates, implements and monitors public policies.

EFFECTIVE POLICIES

In any government structure, irrespective of the country, there are usually strict procedures that establish a policy cycle. Sometimes there is confusion about laws and policies and their differences. The law by its very nature imposes legal requirements on organisations and individuals. A public policy is a way of meeting legal requirements and has to be made within the parameters of the law. Any policy developed, be it by a public organisation or a private childcare centre, must conform to any stated legal requirements.

Public policies differ in how they are expressed, and this can be in many forms, including:

- constitutions
- legislation
- regulations
- statements of belief
- proclamations.

One confusing factor is that policies can be expressed in different ways. However, what does emerge is that policy legitimises decision making. Public policy, then, is much more than a descriptive term, as it involves both process and outcome. It is concerned with the pursuit and achievement of goals.

Economic issues and policy

This aspect (economic) will touch a raw nerve with many early childhood administrators, as the non-compulsory sector has always been vulnerable to government cuts and rationalisation. One might well ask, why is this so?

The most important policy issue confronting governments in both developed and underdeveloped countries is economic policy. However, economic policy is extremely complex in all countries, as it is tied to employment and unemployment, inflation and trade. The market economy, or macroeconomics, influences greatly the kinds of public policies generated by governments. In particular, the economic market affects society in many ways, giving rise to development of compensatory policies for those groups of people in need. Hence, social policies are tied to economic policies, as economic development is very fluid, fluctuating more in some countries than others. The situation requires social policies to be relatively fluid as governments try to compensate for inequalities.

Social policies emanate in various forms, such as unemployment policies, welfare policies, health policies and education policies. These all are tied to the economic base of each particular country. As Fenna (1998: 7) proposes, social policy is inextricably linked to economic policy, and decisions about how best to generate wealth have repercussions on the way wealth is distributed and vice versa. In summary, public policy is continually influenced for better or worse by economic conditions, and comes into conflict with competing demands for resources in order to compensate for social inequalities.

Throughout the world it is recognised that one of the main challenges facing governments, irrespective of their political orientation, is the adequate and equitable allocation of resources. All countries, including the more affluent, have to cope with how to alleviate the social problems—particularly of those people in need. Sound social justice policies focus on fairness in the allocation of resources in accordance with rights, equity and access.

Implementing social justice policies is most difficult in developing countries, where there is a shortage of resources and a plethora of critical problems that often involve the very survival of the people. Over the years we have seen where a lack of policies and lack of government intervention have resulted in large-scale disasters. We are presented with the stark scenario of what happens when countries are ravaged by violence. This also reflects what happens in regimes with an imbalance between coherent social justice policies on the one hand and overactive policies on war and aggression on the other. Sometimes it is easy to see what will happen as the result of a lack of sound social policies. By contrast, the implementation of appropriate, well-planned and carefully developed policies that bring many social benefits to people, and substantially improve the quality of life for a broad spectrum of individuals and society at large, is often difficult for the outsider to 'see'. Sound policy formulation and implementation is fundamental to good government.

Writing of education as a public and private good, Razik and Swanson (2001: 258) propose that:

> *... education brings important benefits to both the individual and society. If public benefits were simply the sum of individual benefits there would be no problem but this is not the case. Frequently there are substantial differences between societal and individual interests.*

This statement certainly describes the current situation in education in Australia, where competing demands cause much debate about the priority and direction of government policies in education. For example, privately run (independent) schools attract government funding comparable to government (state) administered schools. However, as the number of families sending children to independent schools is extremely high in Australia, if the government were to change and/or reverse its funding policy to independent schools, there would not be sufficient places at government schools for the total school-age population. Razik and Swanson (2001: 259) go on to say:

> *Decisions about the nature of education for a society's youth, how it will be provided, and how it will be financed are prime points of interaction. Decisions about public involvement in education are made in political arenas; but the decisions made in those arenas will have strong economic implications for individuals and for private businesses as well as for communities, states and the nation.*

The influence of external forces

There are external forces that influence and/or limit the policy options available to government. These include:

* the economic forces that govern and influence a country's market economy;
* immigration (for example, Australia has been the subject of much controversy in relation to its immigration policies and has had international publicity about this);
* international conventions and agreements, such as the International Convention on the Rights of the Child;
* geographic influences—size and location of a country are important in relation to this factor;
* technological developments and demands;
* defence needs and priorities;
* legal changes (e.g. High Court judgments in relation to land rights judgments in Australia);
* media focus and attention;
* changing demographic patterns;
* interest or lobby groups; and
* social issues (e.g. the environment, education, welfare and health).

Who are the key players in developing public policies?

We have seen from earlier discussion that government is the major force in devising public policy. In democratic societies one would expect the answer to this basic question to be straightforward and that all people had the right/opportunity to be engaged in, or at the very least consulted on, a particular policy that would have a significant effect on people's lives. People affected or likely to be affected by a policy will want to be consulted and to influence the direction and outcomes of the policy. Industrial unions, for example, take an active interest in policies that are likely to affect the employment conditions of their workforce members and will lobby actively for certain positions to be taken.

Around election time one sees a very public display and often debate about a particular government party's policies. It would, however, be fair to say that at election times there is often a discrepancy between an intended policy and what eventuates in reality. In practice, it is the politicians and other government staff who come up with the list of policies they want to carry out if elected to government, at such times often bypassing the important consultation process. Fenna (1998: 13) states that:

> Some policy-making occurs through an exhaustive process of democratic consultation; some gets made through a narrow process of bargaining between dominant interests and some gets made bureaucratically; some emerges as a political gamble; some policy-making begins as an elite exercise conducted behind closed doors but is forced into the open by the mobilisation of other interests.

Zollo, in an external studies guide for the University of South Australia (1998), discusses the work of Colebatch (1998), a writer on Australian policy. She states that Colebatch takes an interesting perspective, proposing that discussions about who makes policy should be focused on trying to identify participants in the process rather than on identifying a narrowly defined group of 'policy makers'. Colebatch suggests that elements of policy making give people a different basis for participating in the policy process, these elements being authority, expertise, and order.

In examining Colebatch's (1998) analysis there are some identified constructs. The first of these is *authority*, perceived to be fundamental and the most obvious basis for the right to participate in the policy process, as policy is about 'authorised decision making'. Who has the authority depends on the details of the specific case. His discussion reveals that authority is in fact 'a construct which frames the world in particular ways' (Colebatch 1998: 17). The relationship between ministers, departmental officials and the Cabinet, for example, is complex. The flow of authority is both top-down and bottom-up. Ministers and Cabinet have authority and others, such as specialist advisers to a minister or experts outside the bureaucracy, seek to establish that right by gaining ministerial approval for submissions or plans. It is evident that authority 'frames the action', in ways that make it easier for some and more difficult for others to participate in the policy process (Colebatch 1998: 18). There have been some recent examples in Australian government policy making—immigration, for example, when departments or other ministries outside immigration have had to feed in information and the efficacy or accuracy of this has been questioned, resulting in government enquiries.

In examining the next construct—that of *expertise*—Colebatch (1998) proposes that policy is also about problem solving. Therefore, having expertise relevant to the problem can be a basis for participating in the policy process. Expertise tends to be specific rather than generic. Within government, designated agencies deal with specific areas of policy. For example, responsibility for education policy rests with education departments. This will be well known to early childhood personnel who are attached to or work for education departments. According to Colebatch, expertise is an important way of organising policy activity. When addressing problems it is essential to know who has special knowledge and where they are located so that the problems can be discussed and expertise shared. It follows that there are links between experts located in government and experts located in other institutions such as universities. Experts then are considered significant groupings in the policy process as perceived by Colebatch.

The third construct proposed by Colebatch (1998: 21) is that of *order*. He writes that 'policy is concerned with making organised activity stable and predictable'. This action involves negotiations among organisations, both government and non-government, as suggested above in the discussion on expertise, who have some responsibility for the policy area. Negotiations are needed and often fraught with difficulty as people with competing demands seek to find common ground.

Bridgman and Davis (1998: 11) propose that the domains of politics, policy and administration interact to produce an agenda for government, assign responsibility for preparing options, and draw up a timetable for Cabinet consideration and implementation. However, policy cannot ignore the 'issue drivers', those external and internal factors that throw up topics for resolution; this of course is what happens, as governments cannot always set the wider policy agenda.

Ways of influencing public policy

From previous discussions on key players it might appear that public policy is far removed from the sphere of influence of families, communities, professionals, interest groups and so on. However, if one understands the process of public policy development and recognises the accountability of politicians to their constituents, then people can attempt to influence policy. From the phases of policy development it can be seen that during the consultation phase a person can make representations either verbally or in written submissions. Public meetings and public consultations are often held and it is in these contexts that people with concern about a policy need to be well prepared, by:

- presenting evidence with reasons well substantiated as to why a certain policy or section of a policy will be detrimental to a public cause. If there is some documented evidence of the problem this should be presented in a professional way. Politicians and policy makers need to be made aware of problems or potential problems;
- gathering supporting or opposing views on the policy from a number of people so that a consolidated response can be presented; and
- presenting a strong advocacy position on some alternative way of dealing with either sections of the policy or the policy itself. A proactive position, clearly documenting an alternative way forward, can be of great use.

If the consultation process has not brought about any suggested changes, it is important to continue to monitor the policy and to suggest that evaluations of the policy be made public.

Politicians should be informed of any ongoing concern that constituents have about certain policies. Governments have been known to amend their policies as a result of advocacy action by various groups, including lobby groups.

Following due process is important when trying to influence public policy by knowing exactly what are the intended processes and time frame. It is difficult to be an effective early childhood advocate, for example, if one does not understand how to influence a policy. In a feature entitled 'Advocacy' in *Rattler* (1999), it is proposed that understanding how law and public policy are developed is an essential first step in effective participation and advocacy. This feature adds that by increasing awareness about how decisions regarding policies and laws are shaped by interest groups and others, advocates have successfully intervened in the policy- and law-making processes.

Policy is a pervasive process

In spite of earlier comments made in this chapter, it seems that many people are concerned with and involved in some form of policy making.

For example, a review of the employment section of the national newspaper *The Australian* on 2 February 2002 showed that many government positions—local, state and national—feature policy as being fundamental to the job description (2002: 21-3):

- A local government shire council advertised for a manager of organisational services, stating that 'the manager is responsible for the development of policies, guidelines and procedures designed to ensure effective and consistent service delivery'. Furthermore, the experience required for this position included significant experience in policy formulation and implementation.
- Another position situated at a state level sought applicants who 'must possess sound understanding of policies, funding opportunities at local, state and national levels'.
- Some positions advertised specifically for policy officers, and had statements in the position description such as: 'The key functions of this position are to give direction and prepare input into the formulation and implementation of policies and sound understanding of policy instruments including legislation'.
- An executive government position sought a person with demonstrated 'capacity for developing high-level policies and demonstrated ability to implement government policies on workplace diversity, workplace participation, and occupational health and safety as applied in the workplace'.
- Some of the positions advertised had role descriptions that specified the required skills. For example, a senior policy adviser was sought who had 'strong well-developed, analytical skills, experience in policy formulation and implementation'.
- Some advertisements were for policy analysts, where the challenge was to develop advice to government ministers with the capability to determine policies.

Governments have become increasingly accountable for the development of sound policies that have the potential to improve quality of life for their citizens. Personnel who work for government obviously must have experience and knowledge of, and commitment to the development of, what are known as public policies.

A review of business and other positions in the employment section of the same newspaper (*The Australian* 2 February 2002) showed little evidence of policy as being fundamental to job requirements. Some business positions sought people with strong managerial skills and knowledge of strategic planning and implementation rather than policy development experience. However, all businesses must function under legislation and are not exempt from reporting requirements. In addition, all businesses have, in some form or other, numerous policies that direct the process of their business. Such policies may or may not be 'public policies'.

PROBLEMS ASSOCIATED WITH THE IMPLEMENTATION OF PUBLIC POLICIES

Some policies have a smooth passage into practice, while others are fraught with difficulties which can be ongoing. There are a number of reasons why policy implementation can be problematic, including the following:

- lack of consultation with stakeholders and relevant interest groups— those most affected by the policy;
- inadequate recognition of the diversity of interest groups. This is particularly relevant in multicultural countries like Australia, Singapore and Hong Kong, where politicians may overlook the complexity of the cultural mix of the population;
- inadequate information being made available about the public policy and its implications;
- resistance or conflict by interest or lobby groups to the policy itself;
- inaccurate interpretation of the policy;
- insufficient lead-time to plan for the implementation process or an unrealistic time frame;
- inadequate planning and development of specific implementation strategies;
- insufficient resources, both physical and human, to implement the policy successfully;
- media pressure or inaccurate or sensational media reporting; and
- lack of opportunities for staff development or retraining of staff affected by the policy.

EXAMPLES OF PUBLIC POLICY

First example: Compulsory Education Act in Singapore

The following policy is an example taken from Singapore, a small, multiracial society of some 235000 people. The Singaporean government proposes that sound policies are essential for achieving social cohesion and national stability. Education policies are important and have impact on the many stakeholders, including children, parents, teachers, principals, professionals and the wider community. A recent policy initiative has been the introduction of the *Compulsory Education Act 2000—Singapore* passed by the Singapore Parliament on 9 October 2000, agreed to by the President on 16 October and to be implemented in 2003 (Gazette no. 27 of 2000). Compulsory education is defined in the report of the Committee of Compulsory Education as:

> ... *education in national schools for Singapore children residing in Singapore, subject to the exemption of certain categories, as a means of further reinforcing the two key objectives of giving our children a common core of knowledge which will provide a strong foundation for further education and training to prepare them for a knowledge-based economy and giving our children a common educational experience that will help to build national identity and cohesion. (Ministry of Education 2000e)*

Background

In 1999 Prime Minister Goh Chok Tong became concerned about some 1500 children (3% of a cohort) in Singapore who were not registered for education in schools. He said 'every Singaporean matters, every Singaporean child should be given the same head start in life, and that is, to attend school' (*Straits Times* 20 November 1999). As a result a committee was set up in 1999 and chaired by the Senior Minister of State Education, Dr Aline Wong, to study the issues relating to compulsory education. The terms of reference of the committee were to consider whether compulsory education should be introduced and, if so, what form and duration it should take (Ministry of Education 2000a). A process of consultation and participation followed as the committee held discussions with interest groups, other community groups, leaders and members of the public. After due discussion, in August 2000 the committee recommended six years of compulsory education (Ministry of Education 2000a).

The *Compulsory Education Act 2000* was legislated with the following goals (Ministry of Education 1999a, 1999b, 2000b, 2000c, 2000d, 2000e):

- to ensure that all children, if possible, attend national schools and benefit from the national education system;
- to give children a common core of knowledge that will provide a strong foundation for further education and training that will give them the competitive edge for a 'knowledge-based economy'; and
- to give children a common educational experience that will help build national identity and cohesion.

Outcomes

- A bigger education budget is to be allocated in order to give the resources needed for implementation of the policy.

- The Singapore government is prepared to enforce various sanctions as stipulated in the Act for non-compliance.
- The Singapore government is prepared to allocate additional resources to cope with truancy and other unforeseen problems relating to the enforcement of compulsory education.
- Children with disabilities are automatically exempted from the policy but they should not be discouraged from benefiting from a national education if desired. Therefore, provisions for integration must be made to accommodate children with disabilities.
- The Ministry of Education will set up a board for compulsory education with representatives from different communities to actively maintain and evaluate the compulsory education policy.
- The Singapore government with the support of its key ministries will strive to educate the general public about the importance and benefits of compulsory education.
- The government of Singapore has initiated a Manpower 21 policy, which is a blueprint to support growth in the knowledge economy and whereby higher-value professional services are to be promoted (http://www.mom.gov.sg/m21/index.htm). The new policy on compulsory education will be in line with Manpower 21.
- A lead-time has been established by government in order to allow for necessary adjustments by all those potentially affected by the introduction of this new policy.

Second example: immigration regulations for foreign domestic workers in Singapore

Background

Singapore is a highly developed country with a relatively wealthy economy. However, government policies recognise that there are limited natural resources available, and human resources are most important. Many Singaporean families employ domestic staff to assist with household duties, thus allowing for maximum participation in the workforce of both men and women. Women's participation in the workforce grew from 28.6% in 1970 to 51.1% in 1997 (Government: Singapore Department of Statistics 1997).

Because of the dependence on foreign workers over the past 20 years in Singapore, the Ministry of Manpower has set up an immigration policy to control the flow of foreign domestic workers into the country. The policy sets out requirements for foreign labour, and different types of permits are issued to regulate the type of work that can be engaged in and levels of payment. The government, by imposing security bonds on employers, reduces concern about population growth of unskilled workers in a country aiming to maintain a high standard of living (Ng, Gan & Menon 2001).

These domestic workers come from neighbouring countries such as Malaysia, Indonesia, Thailand and the Philippines. In order to control the immigration of domestic workers, the Singapore government has implemented a range of measures that employers must conform to when employing a foreign domestic worker.

The policy

The policy determines that a security bond (of Singapore $5000) is paid in order to transfer responsibility to the employer. Permits are granted only after the security bond has been paid. The bond details the duties of the domestic worker and other key elements that must be adhered to.

Outcomes of the policy

- Government is able to control the numbers of foreign workers allowed into the country and the type of work they can legally engage in.
- Government transfers all responsibility for the worker to the employer.
- Employer and employee are to be in mutual agreement on the conditions of the employment.
- The security bond does not, however, protect the rights of the foreign worker, and employers can place restrictions on the worker's liberties.

These examples of policies in Singapore reflect earlier points made in this chapter, that economic developments in a country determine to a large extent the types of policies made and implemented. It is recognised also that national policies affect one another and need to be complementary in their approach. For example, immigration policies affect manpower, economic and political policies.

PUBLIC POLICY FROM THE EARLY CHILDHOOD PRACTITIONER'S PERSPECTIVE

Early childhood personnel have probably been more affected by public policy than any other sector of the education field. In Australia as far back as 1974 they were subjected to federal government policy in relation to so-called 'integrated services'. The then government implemented a policy whereby government funding would be reduced if centres did not immediately adopt an integrated services approach to the delivery of services to clients. This policy required staff to go beyond offering a normal kindergarten program and to introduce additional elements, such as play groups, toy libraries, resource centres, pre-entry groups, before- and after-school-hours care and occasional care.

The non-compulsory sector of early childhood—that is, the services for the 0–5 age group—has always been vulnerable to government funding changes and cutbacks. However, lobby groups and societal changes (e.g. the increased number of women in the workforce leading to greater need for child care) have been trends with a real momentum, and have necessitated the development of new policies.

Specific policy development in early childhood services

The public policy framework outlined earlier in this chapter has significance for early childhood service delivery, whatever form it takes. Without government support and legislation these services would not have the impact needed to meet public demands, they would be too costly for potential users and be without the authority, expertise and order presented as fundamental to policy.

In addition to the public government policies, early childhood services must for their survival as a public service have well-defined, clearly presented policies that are evident in all functions of the services delivery. The following statement, from a director of a childcare centre, on formulating policies is interesting: 'Promoting policies in interesting and imaginative ways not only keeps everyone informed as to what the centre policies are, it also maintains communication between the centre and people who use it' (Magill 1993: 24).

An overarching policy in a particular early childhood service such as a kindergarten would need to include the philosophy, the goals and intent of the service and how these will be realised. It would state the proposed processes and outcomes of the service delivery, including any legal and government requirements. Policy development in an early childhood service will be influenced by:

- the geographic context of the centre, including the physical environment;
- the situation of the service (whether it is part of an integrated services centre, attached to a school, situated in a community centre etc.);
- the client group that uses the service, including the cultural background and needs of families;

- the actual services that are delivered, the range and hours of operation;
- the ages, needs and safety requirements of the children in the service;
- the philosophy and overall role(s) of the service;
- any government department policies or requirements that bind the centre to certain obligations (e.g. curriculum frameworks);
- the training of the staff;
- the numbers of staff, both professional and paraprofessional;
- whether the service has been accredited (e.g. in Australia, by the National Childcare Accreditation Council);
- staff development requirements; and
- occupational, heath and safety requirements for staff working in the service.

From this list, the development of an overall policy for a centre may seem daunting but is an extremely important task. Without it, staff and children are likely to be at risk in one form or another. This does not mean that one can mandate for every action intended or unintended, but it does mean that legal protection for children, staff and families is clearer if a policy is clearly formulated and implemented.

A policy document for an early childhood service should not be confused with licensing regulation requirements, as these are specific and relate to licensing requirements usually under government legislation. Such licensing regulations vary from country to country, also varying within country boundaries or states. They do, in most cases, indicate the minimum requirements for setting up a business or service.

Specific management policies for early childhood services and the early years of school can be looked at from a micro-level. These policies need to be in accord with the public policies of government, but they take on a specific orientation and are geared to the needs of a service.

Overall policies for the children and families who use the services

The following is a list of some of the policies an early childhood service must develop. From the perspective of an individual centre these should be integrated into one policy document and be accessible to all people involved in the centre's activities:

- an overview statement documenting the aims and goals of the service;
- admission and enrolment procedures;
- board of management procedures;
- partnership with parents;

- health policy (including medication, nutrition and safety—this will include accident procedures, immunisation, infectious diseases, medication procedures, 'sun smart', food requirements, menus, rest and/or sleep procedures, permission forms to be filled in by families);
- inclusive curriculum policies, including disability and special needs;
- behaviour management;
- visitors to the service, including students, volunteers and community visitors; and
- excursions and community involvement in excursions.

Policies for staff who work at the service

These will include:

- any information relating to rosters, hours of work, procedures if unable to attend work, lunch and other breaks, procedures in relation to relief staff, staff hygiene requirements;
- industrial requirements, including work hours and conditions of service, sick leave allowances, annual leave and maternity leave, grievance procedures;
- occupational health and safety requirements, accident and injury procedures, occupational rehabilitation;
- reporting requirements to the board of management and any external bodies (e.g. relevant ministries or departments);
- staff meetings and other centre professional commitments;
- staff development;
- information relating to the resources of the service (where the first aid kit is located, where parents are to be interviewed, where staff can go for tea/lunch breaks etc.);
- reporting responsibilities of staff, including forms to be filled in (e.g. when a child has an accident, admission forms, medication forms, excursions, mandatory reporting, permission forms, hot weather policy);
- procedures to be followed in an emergency (e.g. fire);
- curriculum policy and planning procedures;
- communication with families, including policies for bringing and collecting children;
- custody procedures;
- procedures to be followed in relation to the supervision of children, both indoors and outdoors;
- ethical and confidentiality issues;
- student and volunteer placements;

- conflict resolution in the service; and
- a smoke-free workplace policy.

To return to the OECD thematic review, this publication concludes with some pointers for policy makers in relation to addressing some of the problems with policies in Australia's ECEC provision. These are in summary as follows (Hayes & Press 2000: 62):

- the provision of good-quality, affordable and accessible ECEC in the year before school starts;
- addressing the shortage of qualified staff and improvement of staff retention and overall status;
- recognition of the role of early childhood teaching qualifications;
- expansion of culturally responsive ECEC options for indigenous communities to address such problems as those of health and child development;
- enhanced access to ECEC for all children with additional needs;
- ongoing facilitation of continuity between all ECEC settings;
- strengthening of partnerships with parents, communities and ECEC providers;
- development of a comprehensive research base and enhanced ECEC research capacity;
- identification of ECE as a research priority;
- promotion of ongoing dialogue between all relevant government departments concerned with ECEC to develop a national framework;
- development of shared understanding between all relevant portfolio areas and cohesive policy responses;
- evaluation of new and existing ECEC programs in light of outcomes for children in order to provide a better understanding of the implications of policy on the experiences of young children.

These strategies, if addressed by governments in their policy development and implementation, would significantly improve opportunities for the critical years of development of Australia's youngest and most vulnerable citizens.

PROMOTING UNDERSTANDING OF POLICIES

As well as negotiating and finalising policies there is the important factor of promoting awareness of policies, particularly with the parents and wider community. Rodd (1998: 4) states that some of the skills that early childhood professionals need to learn in order to develop into influential policy makers are conference presentation skills, public relations skills for working with/ talking to the media, and writing skills for a range of audiences. This expertise as identified by Rodd (1998) may result in opportunities to participate in policy-making contexts.

Some practical ideas proposed by Elizabeth Magill (1993: 24) for promoting policies are useful. These are that policies can be promulgated through:

- centre and staff handbooks;
- noticeboard displays;
- newsletters;
- parent information sessions—in the evening, on weekends or at other convenient times; and
- staff meetings—staff may also promulgate policies in their interactions and work with parents and the wider community.

EXAMPLES OF SPECIFIC POLICIES OR SECTIONS OF POLICIES RELEVANT TO EARLY CHILDHOOD

The following policies are presented as examples. Each service will need to modify, change and develop from time to time its own policies to suit the philosophy of children and families who use the service, and to meet licensing requirements.

1. Accident policy

The aim of this policy is to ensure that the safety and wellbeing of the child is maintained and that procedures to be followed in the case of an accident are clearly understood by both parents and centre staff. When an accident occurs, the following procedures will be put into place.

- ### *In the case of a serious accident*

  - Get a staff member to call an ambulance or get urgent medical assistance; parents are to be contacted immediately. Stay with the child and render any first aid.
  - In the case of an ambulance being called, one staff member is to travel with the child.

- ### *For accidents that are not deemed emergencies*

  - Administer any first aid if/as needed and render comfort to the child.
  - The first aid kit is located in the sick bay area.

- Check to see whether the other children are being supervised by a staff member.
- Ask a staff member to phone the parents and to clearly explain the context of the accident and the injuries sustained by the child.
- Administer to the ongoing needs of the child and be available to explain the situation when the parent arrives.
- When the child's needs have been satisfied, fill in an accident report form for the parent to witness when he/she comes for the child.
- Explain the accident to all staff so that they are aware of the situation. If the accident has involved equipment or materials, make sure these are removed until the accident has been reviewed by staff.
- In the event that medical attention is required, staff members need to compile a report which should be entered in an accident report book.
- If the child is absent for a time due to the accident, make ongoing enquiries into the progress of the child.

2. Policy relating to children becoming ill while at the centre

The aim of this policy is to ensure that children are supervised and given any attention necessary when they become ill at the centre. However, the policy requires that parents be notified immediately and that arrangements be made by the parents to collect their child as soon as possible.

It is essential that parents accept responsibility to collect and care for their child when they become ill. There are health regulations preventing the centre from keeping a child there, in order to minimise the possible spread of infection to other children.

- *Our procedures*

- When a child becomes ill, he/she is isolated from the other children, taken to a designated section of the centre and made as comfortable as possible.
- A parent is contacted and, if unavailable, the emergency numbers on the admission form will be contacted.
- Ongoing supervision is given to the child, who is reassured that someone is coming to collect him/her.
- In the instance of an emergency, when immediate medical attention is required, a parent will be contacted and the child will be taken by ambulance (if needed) or car for medical assistance to the places identified on the admission form.
- If parent or emergency contacts cannot be reached, approval has been given on the admission form for the director of the centre to act on medical advice at a clinic or hospital.

3. Access-to-children policy

Our centre has a very important and clear policy in relation to child access.
   No child will be allowed to leave the early learning centre with anyone other than the parent or authorised guardian.

- ### *Our procedures*

   Our policy is based on regulations that require:
   - the child to be signed in on arrival and departure;
   - parents to enter details of nominated person/s on the enrolment form and, in addition, to notify in writing if another person is collecting the child;
   - a copy of child custody documents to be lodged at our centre (any change in custody arrangements must be notified to the centre);
   - only persons over the age of 15 to collect children from the centre.

4. Staffing policy

The staffing policy at our centre is in accord with state government child/staff ratio regulations. This child/staff ratio is as follows:

- Children under 3 years—1 staff member allocated to every 5 children.
- Children over 3 years—1 staff member allocated to every 15 children.
- Primary caregiver—with children under 3 years, a primary caregiver allocated who has main responsibility for the care, education and welfare of 5 children.
- Students and volunteers—the centre works with the university and TAFE colleges to assist in the ongoing training of students. Volunteers are also welcome but the number of students and volunteers is closely monitored.

All employees are required to obtain a police check before commencing work with us. This is essential to maintain the safety of all children using the centre.

5. Children with special needs policy

Our centre is pleased to enrol children with special needs, but availability depends on age-appropriate vacancies. Staff are trained to plan and provide a developmentally appropriate curriculum which integrates children with special needs.

It is essential that parents wanting to enrol their child have an informal discussion with the centre coordinator so that an appropriate plan can be devised for the child. All information shared by parents is kept strictly confidential.

Over time it is hoped that children with special needs can be integrated successfully. However, if a child shows an inability to adapt to the centre and excessive demands are made on staff for care and attention, the enrolment will have to be reviewed. If centre management, on review of the child's case study, feel that it can no longer make provision, the parents will be advised of alternative care provision.

- ### *Advice from other professionals*

  With parents' permission, specialised advice may be sought in order to provide for a child's individual needs.

  It is important that parents accept the above policy procedures on enrolment of their child.

6. Outdoor sun safety policy

In order to protect children from the potential skin damage caused by harmful ultraviolet sun rays, the centre adheres to an outdoor sun safety policy.

Children are required to wear hats that protect their face, neck and ears in the outdoor environment. Children who do not bring a hat may be asked to stay indoors.

7. Parental involvement policy

Our centre believes that positive parent involvement assists in the provision of best care and education of the child. Parents are encouraged to:

- spend time in our centre with their children;
- share their talents with the centre;
- engage in two-way discussions with staff about their children's developmental progress;
- share in the program development of the curriculum by contributing ideas in ongoing discussions with staff;
- assist in planned excursions;
- read and respond to monthly newsletters, noticeboards and any other centre communication;
- join parent committees;

- attend and contribute to social and fundraising functions;
- contribute to special curriculum events, such as cultural and festival happenings celebrated at the centre; and
- make use of the centre's toy library and other available resources.

8. Health, medical and safety policy

Our centre operates under a health, medical and safety policy in order to protect all children. Children who are sick will not be admitted to the centre, as the risk of infection to other children may be high. Also, children are best cared for in a home environment if sick. Parents are required to keep their child at home until fully recovered.

On occasion, children will become sick at the centre. In this instance, parents are notified immediately. Children should be collected as soon as possible after parent notification. If sick, the child will be excluded from the group to prevent possible infection of other children. Exclusion of children suffering from infectious diseases is in accord with Health Department regulations. Children can not recommence until a doctor's certificate of health is presented.

• *Medication*

- All medication must be handed over by parents to a staff member.
- Medication must be in an original container with label.
- Written permission by parents must be noted in the medication sign-in book.
- Staff are not allowed to administer medicine if the above procedures have not been followed.
- Staff are required, before administering medication, to have it checked by another staff member, who must also witness its administration to the specific child.

• *When to keep your child at home*

Children should be kept at home if one or more of the following symptoms occur in the previous 24 hours, and parents are encouraged to seek medical advice before children return to the centre:

- vomiting
- diarrhoea
- a fever or temperature of 38°C or above
- rashes or spots
- eye, nose or ear infections
- open or discharging sores
- breathing problems.

9. Mandatory reporting policy

Government legislation states that it is the duty of any centre to report any reasonable suspicion of the following: '. . . a child has suffered or is likely to suffer significant trauma as a result of physical or sexual abuse and that the child's parent or legal guardian has not protected or is unlikely to protect the child from such harm'.

- ### *Sample excursion authorisation*

I give permission for my child, _____, to participate in an excursion on _____ to the zoo at _____.

   Transport is arranged by bus and the cost of _____ is payable on return of this form.

   Children and attending adults are asked to bring their own lunch, which will be eaten in a nearby park.

   Curriculum activities include viewing and discussing the animals, visiting the children's zoo and participating in feeding animals.

   The ratio of adults will be 1 : 10, including two teachers, three assistants and parent helpers.

   I do/do not (circle as appropriate) give my child, _____, permission to attend the excursion.

   Signed _____

   Parent/Legal guardian

- ### *The importance of policies*

Farmer (1995: 7) reminds us of what might happen if there are no written policies. These are, in summary:

- Management may make decisions on the basis of personal opinions, wishes, biases or on an uninformed basis.
- Staff may make the decisions, excluding all other stakeholders.
- Decisions may be referred to different groups within the service who may not have the expertise to deal with them.
- Staff and management may make decisions on an ad hoc basis as these arise.
- Confusion and conflict may arise between staff, staff and families, and staff and management.

The above are the main reasons, but others could be articulated and have indeed been proposed in the context of public policies earlier in this chapter.

CHAPTER SUMMARY

This chapter has attempted to deal with the processes of public policy and policy as applied to early childhood.

- Public policy can be defined as authorised rules and regulations by which organisations and bureaucracies function.
- Policy is a way of shaping actions, and without clear policies (directions) organisations are likely to become dysfunctional or unclear about a course of action.
- Public policy is usually a statement of political priorities and in fact becomes an expression of the political will of government.
- In any country there are external forces that influence and/or limit the policy options available to governments. These external forces include: economic factors, international conventions, geographical influences, technology developments and demands, defence needs and priorities, legal issues, media, interest or lobby groups, and social issues.
- Internal factors such as staff philosophies, overall centre/school philosophy, contextual issues can all affect or limit policy development.
- There are problems associated with the implementation of policies, and these need to be understood and managed.
- Early childhood services have been affected by public policy making, and personnel need to be aware of issues influencing policy in early childhood.
- Finally, some examples of policies were presented.

 Discussion and reflection

1. Go to a dictionary to find out the meaning of the terms public policy, constitution, legislation, and social justice.

2. Consider what would happen in your centre or in a centre you know if there were not a clear policy on what to do when children were ill. Think through the implications of this and how other children and families might be affected.

3. Go to a local newspaper and find an article focusing on a current government policy. Then answer the following.

(a) Who will be affected by this policy?
(b) Who are the stakeholders?
(c) Which level of government has made the policy?
(d) Note down any other contentious issues in relation to this policy: Why is it in the media?

4. Identify one social issue currently confronting your government. Think about some of the debates that this social issue has generated.

(a) Will it result in some change of policy in order to resolve some of the issues being debated?
(b) Who are the stakeholders in relation to this social issue?

5. Identify some of the groups in your home state who are in need of special government provision.

(a) In what ways are these groups marginalised?
(b) What changes in government policies are needed to redress these inequalities?
(c) For what period of time have these groups experienced difficulties?

6. Who are the key players in government in your country or state in relation to developing early childhood policies?

(a) Which portfolio does early childhood fall under—health, education or social welfare? (This is a serious question, as over the years in the states of Australia it has varied greatly.)
(b) Which minister will you lobby if you want some action or policy change?

7. Identify an important policy in early childhood that needs government intervention or change of government policy (e.g. government funding to child care). Discuss this issue with colleagues and decide on a plan of action.

(a) Who can you lobby and how?
(b) What are the outcomes you want to achieve?

8. The issue of immigration is a concern common to many countries of the world.

(a) What do policy developers need to consider when devising or reworking a policy on an issue as problematic and contentious as immigration?
(b) What conventions would policy makers need to work within?
(c) With whom would they need to consult?
(d) What are the ramifications of ineffective policies on immigration?

Chapter **6**

Reconceptualising advocacy in early childhood

This chapter examines the meaning of advocacy in the context of the early childhood field and considers alternative ways of speaking out for young children and their families. The challenges of being an effective advocate for children working with professionals, parents and the wider community are discussed. 'Tool kits' consisting of learnt skills and knowledge, as well as strategies to maximise advocacy efforts, are described. This includes a discussion on the use of action research methodologies. Notions of being a 'children's champion' and a Children's Commissioner are discussed as leadership roles that can facilitate community participation in seeking improvements for children during their early childhood.

 ## Outcomes

At the conclusion of this chapter, the reader should have:

- worked out what advocacy means in the context of the early childhood field;

- developed an understanding of the differences between the role of an advocate and that of an activist;

- a concept of what being a children's champion means;

- developed an understanding of the roles designated to advocates for children in Australia and overseas.

ADVOCATES AND ADVOCACY

The roles of an advocate conjure up images of fighting for a cause or speaking out in defence of a person or persons. This defence could be on an individual basis, such as in the case of defending the rights of a child-abuse victim, or as a collective, for instance upholding the human rights of refugees seeking shelter in another country. Advocacy can also be linked to an issue or concern from a long-term perspective involving people, animals or vegetation. The worldwide movements to save endangered species such as the pandas in China or the African gorillas, and protection of the Amazon rainforests, denote humanity's concern for various life forms. More localised national issues, such as concern about refugee children held in detention centres in Australia (Hydon 2002), symbolise our interest in protecting the rights of minorities in subordinate positions. Advocates or activists are necessary in such instances because there is a perception of injustice and disempowerment of those people at the centre of a crisis. In speaking on behalf of the Real Rights for Refugee Children's action group, Hydon (2002: 7) explained their purpose thus:

> At best, children in detention have experienced high levels of stress; at worst they can be severely traumatised. Specialist services must be provided to ensure that they begin to recover. The long term consequences of neglecting this are frightening and costly. Many of these children will grow up as Australian citizens. Is this how we build the future?

Findings of research, such as the International Leadership Project (ILP), have shown clearly that early childhood professionals in Australia and Finland, for instance, perceived advocacy as one of the key functions expected of leaders in early childhood (Waniganayake & Hujala 2001). There was strong agreement in both countries that it was necessary to advocate on behalf of young children and their families. The Australian early childhood professionals participating in the ILP also highlighted that they must speak out for themselves and advocate for the profession as a whole. Traditionally, child advocacy has been a central theme, a legitimate and unifying code of conduct for early childhood professionals moving into the public domain. However, speaking out about the early childhood profession itself has been neither popular nor acceptable because it might be misinterpreted as being self-seeking and/or militant. Advocacy about and for early childhood professionals is gaining momentum, in part due to increasing public interest in quality children's services.

The correlation of qualified and experienced personnel with excellence in service quality is now well established (e.g. see Doherty-Derkowski 1995; Pence & Moss 1994). During the 1990s much was written about the low status of the early childhood profession (Brennan 1998; Loane 1997; Kagan & Bowman 1997). By putting together information from different countries around the world, it is easy to see that the poor pay and working conditions combined with a poor public image assigned to early childhood professionals contribute to what is a worldwide phenomenon. Public perceptions are socially constructed and culturally driven, and efforts to reconceptualise the public image of early childhood services must begin within the profession.

Advocates and activists

While advocacy may be described as a traditional role adopted by early childhood professionals, being an activist does not carry the same attraction. Activism is generally perceived as being overtly more radical and revolutionary, directly involved with politics and usually concerned with the governance of a state or nation. Activists, in this sense, are perceived as 'ratbags'—fighters or militants in pursuit of political, social, economic or religious causes. They may use aggressive and disruptive strategies to campaign for and promote public awareness about what is usually an inappropriate use of power.

Strategies used by political activists have varied between extreme aggression and non-violent peaceful demonstrations. Contemporary events, such as the attack on the World Trade Center in New York in 2001 and suicide bombers in countries such as Israel and Sri Lanka, are extreme examples of violent political activism. It is therefore not surprising that activism does not sit comfortably either with the early childhood professionals' public image of being 'nice ladies' (Stonehouse 1994) or with the type of work they do with (innocent) young children, which is regarded as a decent, non-aggressive career for women (Petrie 1992).

Advocates and activists are very similar in that their primary objective is to advance a particular case or cause, usually on behalf of a powerless constituency, on an individual or collective basis. Both advocates and activists have strong beliefs and convictions, and are committed to acting as defenders of justice and equity. Accordingly, they have a strong sense of social and political consciousness, and some assume their responsibilities with missionary zeal. They are willing to exert energy, time and resources to elevate an issue to public scrutiny and vigorously agitate for change (Kirner & Raynor 1999). To this extent, advocates and activists are social reformers who advance issues with passion.

It is difficult to distinguish between advocates and activists because both can adopt either peaceful or violent methods to promote a cause. In terms of their sense of identification and involvement with a particular campaign, they can adopt a high or low public profile, and may choose to work alone or with others.

Why invest in early childhood?

The struggle to raise community awareness and obtain public recognition of the importance of investing resources in children and childhood has been a perpetual brief of early childhood professionals throughout history. Politicians kissing babies at election times, declaring that 'children are the future', is a common world-wide phenomenon! Without substantial public pressure such comments are, to a large extent, empty promises—mere political rhetoric, rarely translated into policy or actioned through changes in practice. Indeed, leadership is the theme and the title of the report on the *State of the World's Children 2002* (UNICEF 2002). In the foreword, Kofi Annan, Secretary-General of the United Nations, wrote:

> *Of all the lessons learned in the past decade, the critical role of leadership is perhaps the most important one to take with us into the new century. Leadership is imperative if we are to improve the lives of children, their families and their communities. We must put the best interests of the children at the heart of all political and business decision-making, and at the center of our day-to-day behaviour and activities.   (UNICEF 2002: 2)*

As community leaders, early childhood professionals can promote and exert pressure on governments to acknowledge the significance of early childhood, not only to safeguard children but also to ensure the future wellbeing of all humanity.

Blank (1997: 42) contends that 'leaders understand the role of well-timed reports and data, as well as the value of experts in promoting their cause'. To do this, one needs to keep abreast of current research, collate appropriate data and be prepared to use them strategically. In Australia, the Commonwealth Child Care Advisory Council (CCCAC), which was charged with the responsibility of advising the chief federal politician and the minister responsible for children's services nationwide, acknowledged the vital importance of supporting children's services through better coordination of and accessibility to relevant data and information. In its Report to the Minister, new developments in brain development research, for instance, were summarised, effectively denoting how complex knowledge can be utilised to capture the benefits and promote the early years more broadly (Marriott 2001: 39). This summary is reproduced, with some minor modifications, as Table 6.1.

As can be seen from Table 6.1, the body of knowledge derived through research on brain development supplies us with 'a physiological basis for long-held convictions' pertaining to the key roles played by adults working with young children during early childhood (Marriott 2001: 33). Brain development research also denotes why it is necessary to seek a balance between short- and long-term views of children and childhood—that is, from considering the present (i.e. the here and now) to the future (i.e. as an investment). This balance is an underlying theme in government policy making on early

Table 6.1 Brain development—what have we learnt?

Old thinking	New thinking
• How a brain develops depends on the genes one is born with	• How a brain develops hinges on the complex interplay between one's genes and experiences—'Use it or lose it'
• One's experiences before age 3 have a limited impact on later development	• Early experiences have a decisive impact on the architecture of the brain and on the nature of adults' capacities
• A secure relationship with a primary caregiver creates a favourable context for early development and learning	• Early interactions don't just create a context: they directly affect the way the brain is 'wired'
• Brain development is linear; the brain's capacity to learn and change grows steadily from birth to adulthood	• Brain development is non-linear: there are prime times for acquiring different kinds of knowledge and skills
• A toddler's brain is much less active than the brain of a university student	• By the time children reach age 3 their brains are twice as active as those of adults

Adapted from Marriott (2001: 33).

childhood. An examination of early childhood policy objectives across OECD nations shows ways in which governments have attempted to accommodate prevailing sociocultural beliefs with the economic and political imperatives of governance (OECD 2001: 38). In Australia, for instance, the provision of child care is closely aligned with supporting the needs of parents in the paid workforce. In this sense, reconciliation of employment data and work and family responsibilities pertaining to women in particular have influenced national childcare policy directives (Brennan 1998b). There has been a slight adjustment to this approach more recently, with the 'acceptance of the wider educational and social benefits for 'at risk' children and families' (Marriott 2001: 31).

Evolving roles and responsibilities of early childhood practitioners indicate the strengthening or expansion of our involvement in matters of public interest. In reporting cases of suspected child abuse, for instance, countries such as Australia have introduced legislative mandates to govern professional behaviour to protect children's safety and wellbeing. In principle, safeguarding children's interests and supporting their families are not new areas of responsibility for early childhood professionals. What is different today is the increasing intensity of the demand for concerted public action to uphold children's rights against competing interests of adults. In part, this change in focus is due to wider economic, social and political changes globally affecting the lives of young children and their families.

Burgeoning public interest in brain research has compelled educators such as Puckett, Marshall and Davis (1999) to issue a warning to 'make haste slowly' and not use this knowledge as a quick fix. In contrasting the perils and promises afforded by brain research, they express concern that:

> ... premature interpretation and misapplication of brain based learning may narrow the focus of early childhood care and education to content, producing cookie-cutter programs and interfering with young children's optimal development and learning. (Puckett et al. 1999: 10)

In the current climate, early childhood professionals must therefore ensure not only that they are well informed about brain research but also that they continue to safeguard a holistic approach to child development that is made visible through everyday practices (UNICEF 2002). There is sufficient evidence to indicate a global agreement that government involvement in early childhood, both as an investor and as an interventionist, is critical to redress societal imbalances as well as to complement and support the primary caregiving responsibilities of the family (OECD 2001; UNICEF 2002). Realisation of these objectives requires leadership, community spirit and political will. As 'children's champions', the onus is on early childhood professionals to locate, digest and drive the knowledge base to raise the profile of early childhood and influence the direction of sufficient public resources to the provision of services for young children and their families.

Being a children's champion

Through the advocacy efforts of early childhood professionals as well as international aid organisations such as UNICEF and the Save the Children Fund, much has been achieved to enhance the lives of young children and their families (OCED 2001; UNICEF 2002). The need to continue these efforts has been well established through continuing discussions on the importance of early childhood. Playing a key role as leaders pursuing issues in the public domain, early childhood professionals have adopted the term 'children's champion' (NAEYC 1996) in order to diffuse misunderstandings in the interpretation and use of the terms 'activist' or 'advocate'. The National Association for the Education of Young Children (NAEYC) uses the notion of a children's champion in association with its Code of Ethical Conduct, as noted in the following pledge (1996: 58):

I promise to do all that I can—at work, at home, and as a concerned citizen—to make sure that all children and families have the opportunity to thrive. I will

1. *speak out on behalf of children at every opportunity;*
2. *do something to improve the life of one child beyond my family or classroom;*
3. *hold public officials accountable for making children's well-being and learning a national commitment in actions as well as in words;*
4. *encourage the organisations to which I belong to make a commitment to children and families; and*
5. *urge others to become children's champions.*

The NAEYC's Code of Ethical Conduct has been revised since 1996, but the basic approach captured in the above statement remains. The Association's website now contains a separate window for 'children's champions', with information on government policies and legislation, reports and research that can affect children's services, and discussion papers, as well as NAEYC's position statements on such critical issues as accreditation and violence prevention. Continuous, on-line access to government officials at all levels is facilitated through this website. It provides an easy and efficient avenue for communication with elected representatives and allows input into the legislative processes. Similar on-line methods are used by other early childhood organisations such as the Children's Defense Fund (CDF) (http://www.childrensdefense.org/getinvolved.php).

The CDF is one of the premier children's lobby groups in the USA and requires further exploration (which is beyond the scope of this book). Two of the innovative and successful campaign strategies used by CDF as described by Blank (1997: 43) are briefly included here to illustrate creative possibilities for lobbying:

*   In a doll campaign in Colorado, 'life-size dolls with messages about individual children's needs were placed on the chairs of state legislators'. This action led to successfully obtaining 'millions of dollars in new investments for services to children and families'.
*   A waiting-list roll in Florida consisting of 'the names of 25 000 families who needed child care assistance was placed down the steps of the state capital building to indicate the magnitude of the need for help in paying for child care'.

Blank (1997: 43) goes on to say that 'leaders must strive to develop new ways to get their messages across'. The examples mentioned above reflect the strength of collective wisdom and imagination.

One also does not need to look too far to find startling statistics clearly denoting that, despite the prosperity of contemporary living standards, there are children whose lives are continually at risk. Raban (2000: v) is resolute in declaring that:

> *... there can be no doubt that early childhood education and care must rise to the top of the political agenda as a way of cherishing and valuing the present, and safeguarding the future. Without this determination, we will be squandering precious human resources.*

TOOLS OF A CHILDREN'S CHAMPION

Jensen and Hannibal (2000: 6) argue cogently that early childhood professionals must actively engage in the public arena now, and that 'the time is right for action' (2000: 5). They declare that individuals must choose between being active or passive proponents of early childhood. They [we]:

> *... can remain part of the advocacy problem, bogged down in helplessness and disillusionment, or we can become part of the solution by coming to grips with substantive issues in the field and obtaining, concurrently, the skills and dispositions needed to become effective advocates. (2000: 5)*

However, the appropriateness of advocacy and activism must be assessed against the local context in which early childhood professionals live and work. Strategies that may be appropriate in one country, setting or state may not be relevant or timely in another. In embracing the role of children's champion, early childhood professionals therefore need to equip themselves with the necessary tools or means of effecting change. Such a 'tool kit' is a mixed bag of personal attributes and learnt skills and knowledge, and may include the following.

Content knowledge

Before one can speak out on any matters one must be knowledgeable about the topic, the content and the key concerns, and their significance for the constituency being defended—be this children or adults. Research undertaken with early childhood practitioners in Australia and Finland also highlighted the importance of understanding the historical context and pedagogical basis of early childhood when speaking out as leaders (Waniganayake & Hujala 2001). This type of background information accumulated over time can enhance the formulation of appropriate and effective strategies. Such an approach is akin to driving a car, keeping one's eyes on the rear-vision mirror while moving forward simultaneously.

Operational context

Awareness of how the system works is a necessary first step in promoting change. Studies about governance—whether about running a local preschool or a childcare centre, or learning about government regulations—are never popular in early childhood training courses. As such, legislative matters are dealt with in an instrumental manner, rarely moving beyond an understanding of their basic accountability requirements. Familiarity with policy-making procedures as well as stakeholder involvement is critical to achieving success as an advocate.

Communication skills

Interacting with other people through verbal and/or non-verbal means is a prerequisite for fostering interest, enquiry and for implementing change in practice. Of particular interest to the children's champion is one's ability to capture media attention, to use it to promote public awareness and to activate debate about children's concerns in the wider community. Identifying and cultivating journalists who are interested in and respectful of children as citizens, and who will therefore provide media access and coverage of issues, can be critical to the success of a campaign for children. Early childhood professionals can also provide active leadership to build alliances across the community, incorporating diversity through dynamic networking and negotiating skills.

Personal disposition

Incorporating temperament and personality traits, one's disposition reflects one's attitudes towards particular issues. When speaking or acting out as a children's champion, one's disposition is on display and is evaluated by others as being appropriate and relevant to the task. Describing it in terms of 'emotional literacy', Jensen and Kiley (2000: 116) state that one's disposition is critical in the formation of a community of learning. Thus, one's beliefs and values can have a significant bearing on the behaviour, argument and logic used to explain the stance adopted by a children's champion. To succeed as an advocate or activist one must make a commitment in time and energy and must also overcome 'feelings of powerlessness and anxiety about anticipated and unanticipated consequences' (in Jensen & Hannibal 2000: 5).

Strategic planning

The importance of selecting the appropriate means of effecting strategic change cannot be underestimated. Having a plan of action begins with the establishment of specific targets or goals and the consideration of methods or strategies to achieve these goals. The pursuing of set objectives will engage the early childhood professional in problem-solving and decision-making processes. The approach taken or the tactics used to convey one's message as a children's champion is dependent on a number of factors, including the topic/issue being defended, time and resources available, as well as the skills and attributes of the advocates themselves. This approach can be seen as an effective use of the research skills acquired during initial training by early childhood professionals.

The way in which all these aspects come alive when one works as a children's champion is beautifully illustrated in Gabby's story. For nearly 25 years, Gabrielle Fakhri has been working to support children and families of immigrant, refugee and asylum-seeker backgrounds wanting to live in Australia. Recently Gabby shared her experiences with us, and the following excerpt is an edited version of a much longer interview.

Gabby's story — responding to refugees and asylum seekers

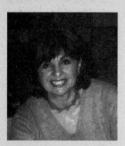

GABRIELLE FAKHRI
Family & Children's Services Program Coordinator
Victorian Cooperative on Children's Services for Ethnic Groups (VicCSEG)
Melbourne
Australia

1. You are currently working with refugees and asylum seekers. What are their primary needs in relation to their children?

I greet people who come off the buses from detention centres in Woomera, Port Hedland and Curtin. One of their main needs is material aid—clothing and food to start with, then furniture, bedding, kitchen utensils and toys. Obviously housing is a major concern. We have to help find them housing. Then they have to furnish the houses on the little income they get from the government. I collect material aid, sort them and get them ready for distribution. I do this work after hours, during the weekends, as a volunteer. It's time-consuming and is now taking a toll on my health and my family life. It's my passion, but I need to get more people to help.

2. Having devoted a good part of your career to advocacy for young children and their families, what are some of your career highlights?

One of my main achievements was setting up the bilingual-bicultural Lebanese child care centre. It took 2–3 years of lobbying and fighting and at the time there

Continued

was a lot of negativity towards me in particular. It was seen as setting up a ghetto for Arabic speakers: it was said that these children were never going to be able to integrate, as they would not speak good English. I had people fighting me at meetings. I cut my teeth on that project. I worked with very wonderful women—especially the Mother Superior, who was the director of the childcare centre. She couldn't speak English so she pushed me into being demanding, so I would go and demand on their behalf. I was their voice. She said that we have a need in our community for our preschool children; they have a right to speak their mother tongue and keep their culture, and we demand child care for them. Now, 15 years down the track, the centre is doing very well. We have a waiting list of 100 and users of every nationality—Greek, Italian, and Christian and Moslem. It has never had just Arabic speakers or Lebanese families.

I've also just set up a Community Resource Centre for Asylum Seekers in a house given to me by the Lebanese community—my people. I first used this place to store the donations we collected. Then the needs of the asylum seekers grew and grew and we had to look at other options. I want this to be a one-stop shop for asylum seekers. I don't want to reinvent the wheel or do it alone. What we're doing is getting all the specialist agencies, like trauma counselling and legal aid, to come into our centre to work with the asylum seekers. For example, one agency is giving us one day a week to process legal issues; Centrelink (the government social security agency) will come one day a week to run information programs; and computer-training classes and English classes are being provided by other agencies. We coordinate the times and programs. It's not ad hoc; it's providing a range of services under one roof. We facilitate access between the people in need and the agencies that can support them. It's a good model for outreach work—a lot of networking and knowing who's who.

3. What are some of the difficult aspects of your work?

Every now and then you get people who are not happy with anything you do. For example, finding cheap accommodation is not easy. It's not my responsibility to redefine or prioritise people's needs. I could meet some of their material needs but their priority may be housing or to locate another family member, a mother or a husband. No matter what else you do, you can't meet that need. It's taken me a while to understand this. I have to be honest and say, 'I know you want this, but I can't help you with that; I can only do this' etc. I'm lucky because in my day job at VicCSEG there is great flexibility and understanding by my colleagues. My paid job involves working with refugee families to meet their childcare needs. But once you establish this contact, you get caught up with their other needs, from housing to clothing to paying bills. It's very hard to back off or refer them to others even when it's outside your area of expertise—like legal aid issues. If you don't support them at that stage, you get a bad reputation and lose credibility. But you have the difficult task of explaining to your funding body that some of these real needs are outside your funded community role. It's not enough to just do the childcare arrangements. It doesn't mean much. We need a more holistic approach to families. That's what's missing, and that's my goal for the community centre that we've set up.

Continued

4. Do you believe there is a difference in being an advocate and an activist in early childhood?

That's a tricky one. Advocacy for me is the more polite way of doing things. It's about talking and talking but you don't really get anywhere. It's like me saying I want to advocate for cheaper child care. If you want to get somewhere, you have to become an activist. As I've grown older I've become more passionate and demanding. I do more of the demonstrating and standing outside yelling, signing petitions and being very vocal. I'm at a stage in my career where I don't worry about the dangers to myself. I find that the polite way of doing things is not working. You need to scream and yell, and I think that comes under activists! To me, an advocate writes nice letters and talks politely. An advocate in Italian is a solicitor and I see that image when I'm writing a letter on someone's behalf, speaking to a childcare centre to make arrangements for a child. But to get change, you have to go the extra yard. You also must have a smile on your face to win people. To be an activist you need to be much more active than an advocate.

5. What are some of the difficult decisions you've had to make in your career?

One of the difficulties is learning to work across diverse cultures. While I'm very comfortable with Arabic-speaking people, my own Lebanese people, it's always hard to establish credibility with other groups. It's a struggle. I've struggled with various communities about difficult issues like domestic violence and incest, and started to form negative views. Something I try not to. When I have realised what was happening to me, I have backed away from that community to reassess how I could work with them again.

With another refugee community the women were very strong and very demanding, and they wore me out! Having been refugees, these women had learnt to be assertive, fighting for their lives and protecting their children. I realised these women were a different type of refugee because they had been in camps all over the world for over 10 years. I admire them greatly but I struggled a lot at first in meeting their demands. It was a matter of my reading up on and getting to know more about their culture and experiences. I also worked with a good interpreter and a key man from that community. I spent a lot of time with them, becoming acculturated and better informed about their community. This took a while, and you do need that time to establish connections.

6. In daring to be different, who has supported you?

My husband. Other people have also noticed this—that he has been my biggest support. He has absolute faith in my work with refugees and asylum seekers. He looks after my children so that I can continue with my voluntary work. Sometimes they come with me. For example, when people donate clothing etc. my extended family—my sisters, nieces and nephews—they are all there in my house, cleaning and sorting through clothes, toys and furniture; it just takes a phone call. It's a big job. I couldn't do any of this without my family's support. My colleagues at work at VicCSEG have also been enormously supportive—never once have they begrudged the time I spend attending to the voluntary commitments that come in at all odd hours.

Continued

> **7. How can early childhood professionals respond to the needs of children from refugee backgrounds?**
>
> I did a training session for about 100 early childhood professionals last week. I was amazed how little information they had about refugees. We need to be better informed—to know where refugees come from, what they have been through and what impact this could have on their children. I had a phone call from a childcare worker who said 'I've got a refugee mother here'. When I asked what country she came from, she replied 'Oh, one of those Middle East countries'. She didn't know the country, the language, the religious background. I would assume there would have been some documentation on this family. I'm shocked that they don't have basic knowledge about families in their centres. In high refugee-intake areas you also need to get in specialist advice from agencies such as the Trauma Counselling Centre to learn what to look for and prepare staff for the impact it may have on them. I'm working closely with the Free Kindergarten Association's Multicultural Resource Centre (MRC). We do tag-team training: I provide information about ethnic backgrounds to facilitate refugee families to get *to the door* of the childcare centre. Then MRC takes over in helping centres to respond to meet needs *inside* the centre. This is a very good combination of expertise.

ADVOCACY TIPS

Children's champions can work individually or align themselves with others to build a coalition and speak with one voice as an organisation or collective. Novice practitioners in particular can benefit from joining professional organisations and working with more experienced others to acquire skills, such as how to deal with the media (when doing a radio or television interview) and to write submissions to public enquiries, including collecting and analysing research-based evidence to support claims.

In their book on advocacy and leadership matters, Jensen and Hannibal (2000: 220–1) offer a range of strategies, formats and helpful hints to guide public scrutiny and debate on issues concerning young children and their families. They present some useful advocacy tips, and these are modified and extended in Figure 6.1.

In Australia, during government election times, there is usually a flurry of activity in the early childhood field. The National Association of Community Based Children's Services (NACBCS) was first established in the 1970s as an outcome of political campaigns to put child care on the federal political agenda (Brennan 1998a). That campaign saw the realisation of the first national Child Care Act being proclaimed in 1972, and the Association has since continued to define the pathways for federal government's involvement in childcare matters. The NACBCS tradition of campaigning for better children's services continues to date, although the militancy of its activists has been somewhat subdued in more recent elections. A lobby kit has been

Figure 6.1 Advocacy tips.

- **Be articulate.** Whether making a written proposal or an oral briefing, early childhood professionals must be able to communicate their messages with conviction in a concise manner, clarifying concerns locally. Identifying three key points to emphasise can help overcome limitations of time and words allocated to convey the message.
- **Be adamant.** Perseverance and patience are the cornerstones of successful lobbying. Once a commitment has been made, it behoves the early childhood professional to remain resolute and seek resolution. Of course, the means used do not necessarily justify the goals in all cases, and use of violence for instance requires careful consideration of the consequences for others as well as oneself.
- **Be constructive.** It is easy to criticise but more effective to offer alternatives to redress imbalances or injustice. Offer lateral solutions to everyday common problems, and develop cost–benefit analysis to strengthen the arguments being presented. Everyone wants to know how to save dollars while saving the world!
- **Be appreciative.** On completing data collection, good researchers always leave the door open for another to be made welcome at the same site. Similarly, children's champions must acknowledge contributions of others, irrespective of defeat or success during a campaign. Sending flowers or dedicating public accolades to all who supported the campaign, including media personnel, ministerial advisers and parent volunteers, is not merely good manners but sensible practice. The goodwill generated will reap rich rewards from a long-term perspective.

Adapted from Jensen & Hannibal (2000: 220–1).

developed and is a regular feature of the NACBCS campaigns, usually containing items such as those shown in Figure 6.2.

The NACBCS campaign kit also explains the need for and importance of lobbying by linking these to the overall goals and objectives of the organisation's own position statement on children's services. During the 2001 federal elections NACBCS also established a website dedicated to its 'Children First' campaign. Visitors to the site were invited to sign up for the campaign by completing an electronic survey. The newness of such strategies may constrain their effectiveness. Having access to on-line infrastructure is not in itself sufficient to run a political campaign. Accordingly, those people and organisations interested in pursuing web-based strategies for lobbying purposes must allocate sufficient time and resources not only to publicise the system but also to educate prospective users and evaluate its effectiveness as a lobbying tool.

Familiarity with key terms in the legislative procedures of one's own country is a prerequisite of political activism. Knowledge about structures of government, the passage of legislation, as well as timelines allocated for debate and discussion, are vital in effecting change through legislative means: 'Although the process usually is lengthy, advocates must be prepared to mobilize on short notice, just in case something moves quickly' (Goffin & Lombardi 1988: 91). Technology, including mobile phones, e-mail and facsimile machines, is an invaluable asset in circulating information, coordinating action

Figure 6.2 Contents of a lobby kit for a public action campaign.

- **Postcards** and **proforma letters** addressed to politicians and **posters** for public display, each containing key points of the campaign expressed succinctly
- **Petition formats** to inform and involve people through signed commitments; can provide tangible expressions of support and symbolise the effectiveness of a campaign
- **Contact lists** for politicians and media to use as appropriate, including arranging visits to centres or invitations to speak at a public meeting. These lists need regular updating
- **Bumper stickers** and **bookmarks** with the campaign theme and contact details for more information
- **Organisational position statements** on campaign issues to achieve consistency in the approach adopted by members
- **Research evidence** to support claims, including statistical data (e.g. changes in government expenditure) and analysis of party political policies on children's services, presented as non-partisan summaries and enabling readers to draw their own conclusions with ease
- **Anecdotal evidence or stories** of disadvantage and hardship from local communities to illustrate points being raised in the campaign; extracts of conversations, quotes and cartoons, for instance, can be used to convey messages imaginatively

Modified from NACBCS (2001).

and planning strategies efficiently and expediently. Systems of communication such as group e-mails or a telephone tree (Kirner & Rayner 1999: 51) should be set up and tested before a campaign in order to maximise their potential during the campaign. As Kirner and Rayner (1999: 52) state:

> Once politicians stood on soap boxes or on the back of trains visiting remote towns to get their messages across. Now the messages can be sent faster and better in new ways. The old principles apply to new methods: get accurate information out fast!

There is little doubt that campaigns for young children and their families provide a catalyst for community action. At the conclusion of a campaign, it is necessary to:

- identify and count up what was achieved;
- assess the losses;
- discuss impediments that may have hindered progress;
- make recommendations for future campaigns; and
- publicise achievements, and celebrate!

The need to rejoice and remain optimistic is highlighted by Crompton (1997: 53), who declares that optimism is an essential attribute to being able to lead and inspire. Even if not much is achieved during a particular campaign, Crompton states that optimists will see this as 'work-in-progress' and 'applaud the incremental changes in the field'. Lessons learnt from each experience are invaluable in moving on and designing the next campaign. When well coordinated, the adoption of a comprehensive lobbying strategy can also assist in the formulation of a nationwide campaign. If the campaign was initially linked to a government election, what began as a campaign with a limited tenure can in the long run provide the infrastructure for a large-scale political movement for children and families. One day we may even see an early childhood professional being elected as a politician, and going on to win portfolio responsibilities as the chief minister responsible for national children's services.

PROFESSIONAL REFORM THROUGH ACTION RESEARCH

Early childhood professionals, when acting as children's champions, must be cognisant of the social construction of their personal beliefs, values and attitudes, and how these factors can influence their professional and political consciousness. Likewise, ideology can blind enquiry through subjectivity. As Kincheloe (1993: 188) puts it:

> ... we learn that all seeing is selective, filtered by the ways that power has constructed our subjectivity. We learn that we see from particular vantage points in the web of reality, coming to realise that there is no value neutral way of perceiving.

It is therefore important to consider alternative ways of engaging in enquiry.

Systematic, research-based enquiry has been traditionally contained within the early childhood academy, regarded as a scholarly activity beyond practitioners such as preschool teachers and childcare staff (Rodd 1994; Takanishi 1986). Today the importance of research-based evidence is taken for granted, yet the challenge of selecting appropriate tools for research remains. Rodd (1994), who believes that leadership is inextricably tied to research, concurs that action research offers a way forward, particularly for early childhood practitioners. It is an appropriate 'vehicle for increasing professionalism because, through the process of conducting action research, practitioners begin to value research and develop a professional culture that values reflection' (Whitford et al. 1987, cited in Rodd 1994: 144).

Given the burgeoning numbers of university-trained early childhood professionals working in preschools and childcare centres, it is argued that these graduates can and should play a central role in conducting research. Small-scale action research projects, for instance, have the potential to transform practices and strengthen the leadership potential of neophyte early childhood professionals. It is a methodology that requires the same people to adopt simultaneously the dual roles of participant and researcher. This is where the notion of 'teacher as a researcher' was first conceptualised (Peltonen & Halonen 1998). Thus, by its very nature, action research offers one of the best strategies of empowerment because it is a system of collective enquiry that involves everyone in thinking, designing, implementing and evaluating the whole process.

The basic steps or phases of the evolution of an action research project are depicted in Figure 6.3. As can be seen, they follows a cyclical pathway where reflection leads to action, and these processes occur throughout the project's lifetime. In effect, action research emulates a journey of discovery learning (Dewey 1933; Schon 1988) actively manipulated by the participants. When managed well, it can enhance the productivity of the enterprise and the practitioners' professional development (Peltonen & Halonen 1998). Realisation of these high ideals is dependent on numerous factors—especially leadership, as well as commitment, tolerance, time and available resources.

Figure 6.3 Doing action research.

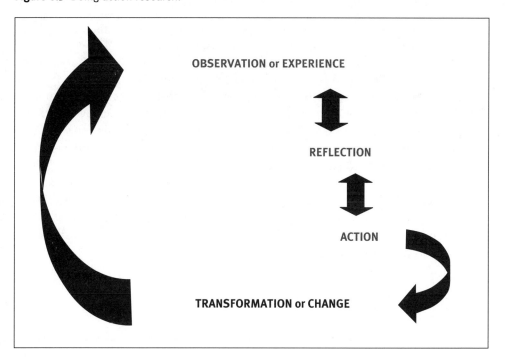

It is not unusual to think that action research offers exciting possibilities, especially for early childhood practitioners who want to remain at the coal-face working with children and at the same time want to carry out research at their centres. The characteristics of action research that are enticing to these professionals include that it is:

- context-specific—making the work directly relevant and meaningful;
- participatory—involving collective and consultative decision-making;
- transformative—with systematic evaluation leading to knowledge creation.

These same dimensions may also be perceived as the weaknesses of action research: that is, being context-specific, the ability to generalise and validate the findings is limited. The notion of participatory decision making is not always easy to implement, especially in hierarchically constructed enterprises where the centre director or the management committee has veto powers. The extent of skills and knowledge gained through the action research process needs to be assessed from a long-term perspective. It is difficult to find studies in early childhood that have attempted to do this systematically. The following comments by Peltonen and Halonen (1998: 90) are pertinent here:

> In the contexts in which all the participants are adults, the systematic use of a discourse based on equality and openness can perhaps be justified in theory and practice. But, it could be asked, what would a discourse or dialogue based on equality mean in research carried out, for example, in kindergartens or day cares, where the majority of the participants are young children?

In other words, how can early childhood practitioners, being participants and researchers in the same project, give voice to the children at their centres?

According to Kincheloe (1993: 188), 'action research conceived within a critical post-modern system of meaning turns inquiry into a higher order cognitive activity'. There is an expanding body of literature on action research involving educationalists as well as other social scientists. It is highly recommended that early childhood professionals acquire, as a basis, a sound knowledge and understanding of the theoretical and methodological considerations of action research. This basis is essential before undertaking action-type research so that the professionals themselves can evaluate the best way to proceed in meeting their specific goals and objectives.

SHARED RESPONSIBILITY

An examination of the national policies across 12 OECD countries has shown a significant policy shift globally, where early education and care is now perceived as 'a shared responsibility between the family and the state and not just for the family alone to bear' (OECD 2001: 40). At the micro-level, practitioners working in children's services also need to recognise the implications of this policy shift for their day-to-day work. Learning to work cooperatively with more knowledgeable others is a fundamental learning strategy not restricted to early childhood (Raban 2000). Working with others is effective, not only because in doing so it provides insight into another person's world of work but because it also expands one's own options and ability to consider alternative ways of doing the same tasks or responding to similar problems. Opportunities to interact and exchange ideas, question each other and reflect together in drawing up plans for action can be deeply empowering experiences.

Kagan and Rivera (1991: 52) have defined collaborations as 'those efforts that unite and empower individuals and organisations to accomplish collectively what they could not accomplish independently'. Responsibilities when shared with others provide authentically holistic learning experiences (Jensen & Kiley 2000: 92). The organisational context of a preschool or childcare centre or the community itself becomes the resource, a platform for knowledge creation. The leadership of early childhood professionals can ensure that the centre becomes a hub for community action and celebration of achievements for young children and their families. Kagan (1994: 53), however, issues a cautionary note by alerting us to consider the *limitations* of shared leadership, as follows:

> Shared leadership is not a panacea. It takes far more resources (time and money) than direct leadership. Not only does shared leadership take time, but it also demands the refinement of skills often taken for granted: communication, negotiation, conflict resolution and empowerment. Sharing leadership demands training that many early childhood leaders have not routinely received via conventional training programs, despite the profession's commitments to it.

A Children's Commissioner

The idea of a Children's Commissioner symbolises the notion of a children's champion in practice. It is also a position of power—a legislative instrument vested with civic responsibilities. As Kirner and Rayner (1999: 3) assert, 'one of the greatest mistakes women can make is to assume that good intentions and hard work will be rewarded. They won't! You need power to make a difference'. The concept of a Children's Commissioner has been explored by many countries and states but implemented by few. It is usually associated with the United Nation's Convention on the Rights of the Child. A Children's Commissioner who has statutory powers of governance is perceived as a tool or a mechanism used by governments to implement the UN Convention.

Norway established the world's first Children's Commission in 1981, as an ombudsman's office. Children's Commissioners can now be found in places such as:

- Sydney, Australia (http://www.kids.nsw.gov.au/);
- Brisbane, Australia (http://www.childcomm.qld.gov.au/);
- British Columbia, Canada (http://www.childservices.gov.bc.ca/);
- London, UK (http://www.londonchildrenscommissioner.org.uk/);
- New Zealand (http://www.occ.org.nz/aboutus/);
- Norway (http://odin.dep.no/odinarkiv/norsk/dep/ud/1999/publ/032005-990429/index-dok000-b-f-a.html);
- Sweden (http://www.bo.se/eng/engelsk.asp);
- Wales (http://www.childcom.org.uk/).

Although this is not a comprehensive list, it illustrates that it is possible to have more than one Children's Commissioner in the same country. In Australia there have been many calls to establish a national Children's Commissioner (Marriott 2001). Due to various factors, including difficulties in obtaining a national commitment in funding, some states such as Queensland and New South Wales have resolved to establish a state-based commissioner in their own geographic jurisdictions.

An examination of available websites for Children's Commissioners as noted above reveals similarities as follows:

- Protecting the best interests of children is their number 1 priority.
- Coverage includes children and youth up to the voting age.
- They are administratively linked to the ministry responsible for children and youth affairs.
- They are an independent public office, separated from government and politically neutral.
- Key functions include child protection and justice, advocacy and public education.
- They represent children in adult forums, through either direct or indirect participation.

An important feature of this public office is its strong commitment to actively demonstrate child-centred practice at all levels of the Children's Commission's activities. This approach is made explicit, for instance, in the Norwegian Children's Commissioner's vision statement, which consists of three key aspects:

1. Children are viewed as equals to adults.
2. Children are regarded as competent individuals.
3. Opportunities will be a focal point when working with children.

The establishment of an 'Internet Parliament' for children in Norway, for instance, reflects another way of empowering young people to engage in discussions leading to voting on child-related policies through mini-referendums. While such initiatives to systematically obtain 'children's and adolescents' opinions have hitherto been rare' (UNICEF 2002: 15), we must be mindful that such efforts 'must be seen not simply as an educational exercise for the children and adolescents involved (as is often the temptation) but as important democratic institutions in their own right' (UNICEF 2002: 16).

The importance of promoting and modelling child-centred practice was also emphasised by Moira Rayner (2001), the first director of the Office of the Children's Rights Commissioner for London. She and her staff were inter-viewed and appointed by an advisory board consisting of children aged 7–15 years. She also described the way in which the meetings of the advisory board were made 'child-friendly', beginning with games and chocolates, and being contained within one hour. Rayner spoke passionately about engaging children directly in the decision-making processes that affect them (Article 12) and the importance of upholding children's basic right to play (Article 31). She lamented that to a large extent, in contemporary Western societies in places such as London, adults' priorities override children's needs and interests. Until adults really learn to listen and allow children to voice their concerns, we will continue to break the UN Convention on the Rights of the Child; it then will remain merely a set of lofty ideals or prin-ciples, read and debated but never truly tested in practice. Collaboration between early childhood professionals and Children's Commissioners can strengthen the profession's obligations to children, both nationally and globally.

How can we translate trust that is anchored in personal relationships to trust in strangers, and move from sociability to civility? One way is to focus not on the individual but on the whole society, by targeting the local communities and not the single child. There are difficulties with this proposition too because the notion of communities is also changing, so much so that citizenship is no longer tied up with holding the passport of one country. Today's families are also highly mobile, and are sometimes described as the 'dot-com generation', prepared to travel and work anywhere, any time. Therefore we need to find new ways of learning to connect with each other. Human beings are essen-tially social creatures, and our survival has always been dependent on being able to relate to others of our species.

Unfortunately, we are moving away from the traditional notion of service to humanity to a new focus that emphasises service to the individual. We are less concerned about collective responsibilities to our children, because of our preoccupation with finding ways to satisfy individual needs and interests. This separation of the individual from the group begins within the family context, and collectively affects the whole society. To redress this pattern of social destruction we have to reflect on what those things are that matter most to each of us. In other words, we have to decide on what it is that we all share, have in common, and want for each other. These are the forces that bind us as human beings (Cox 1995). They consist of:

- trust—goodwill and having faith and belief in someone;
- reciprocity—meaningful relationships or connections. Traditionally, reciprocity was based on kinship ties, which continue to be important in some Asian and African societies;
- mutuality—that is, having something in common or sharing something and being able to rely or count on it;
- cooperation—that is, forming alliances or collaborating to achieve something together;
- time—which is highly valued but is in short supply. We need to find better ways to manage time.

Cox (1995: 5), a leading Australian social activist, states that taken together these five forces build 'social capital', which is the critical mass that is necessary to build a truly civil society. The term social capital, coined by the American social scientist Robert Putnam (1995), is now being used by politicians and policy planners around the world. Social capital is about people's commitment to work collaboratively with others for the common good. Social capital is, in monetary terms, FREE!

It is important that early childhood educators, as human services professionals, engage in this dialogue and learn the talk, and become able to 'walk the talk'! Social capital refers to:

- human interactions or relations between people—it is essentially human behaviour, and requires more than one person to activate; it is dynamic and can change over time;
- participation in networks or groups—as in clubs and voluntary organisations. There is an assumption that it will lead to the creation of stronger social bonds or alliances;
- sharing of resources, time and energy—the participation and contribution make the processes mutually beneficial (Cox 1995; Putnam 1995).

To put it simply, social capital is about learning to live together with others. The net result of creating social capital means that it will not only enhance the social wellbeing of a community but also ensure its economic prosperity. This dual benefit makes the creation of social capital an attractive proposition for everyone. Instead of becoming casualties of change, early childhood professionals can be empowered to take charge of change by sharing their professional knowledge with others. This cooperation leads to the creation of social capital within the early childhood profession. As children's champions, early childhood professionals cannot abdicate their responsibilities regarding the socialisation of the next generation, especially to technology and the media. Instead, as trusted adults, professionals must accept their responsibility for moral education during early childhood. This action is possible if professionals can visualise public- or community-based institutional settings such as preschools and childcare centres being involved with broader social and civic agenda that go beyond the traditional sphere of service delivery in care, education, health or welfare.

The professional's goal must be to create sustainable communities. Professional leadership is essential to make this happen, and to do it effectively early childhood professionals must accept their social and civic responsibilities. This acceptance is necessary for at least two good reasons: first, to enhance the quality of life globally for everyone, children and adults; and second, to achieve unity within diversity so that we may build peace and rejoice in celebrating our differences. Creating sustainable communities requires commitment—a willingness to try, and a drive to succeed. Early childhood professionals, as leading human services personnel, can make that difference.

CHAPTER SUMMARY

This chapter has attempted to examine important concepts of advocacy and activism. It has:

- discussed why advocacy is extremely important to the future status of early childhood;
- explained the thrust of a 'children's champion' approach;
- discussed the advocacy tools of a 'children's champion';
- presented an interview with a family and children's services program coordinator who works with refugees and asylum seekers in Australia;
- presented advocacy strategies for professionals to consider;
- discussed professional reform through action research; and
- presented some advocacy positions, including that of a Children's Commissioner.

 Discussion and reflection

1. What sort of society do you want to belong to, and how can you make a difference for a child every day?

2. Eva Cox has spoken about forces that bind us. How can we translate this knowledge to strengthen the early childhood profession?

3. Look at the following list of strategies a children's champion could use, and reflect on the following questions:

    (a) What acts have you done and/or are you willing to do?
    (b) What are the probable consequences of doing these acts in your country?
    (c) What strategies would you use to maximise the impact of your work either as an advocate or an activist?

    Would you . . .

    - sign a petition?
    - write a letter to a politician?
    - write a letter to a newspaper?
    - march in a political demonstration?
    - be interviewed by the media—newspaper, radio and television?
    - speak at a rally?
    - help organise any of the above?

Chapter 7

Creating the context for conflict resolution in the workplace

This chapter is concerned with the nature of conflict generally and how conflict occurs in many contexts. Early childhood services are not exempt from their share of conflict and, in this respect, identification of the skills and knowledge needed to effectively manage and resolve conflict is discussed. An understanding of the organisational culture of early childhood and sources of possible tension, conflict, stress and burnout is also presented. Options for dealing with the above are examined, including how mediation can be used to negotiate and implement some strategies for resolving disputes.

Outcomes

At the conclusion of this chapter, the reader should have:

- developed an understanding of the nature of conflict;
- a better understanding of the reasons why conflict occurs in early childhood centres;
- the ability to identify conflict and the sources of it;
- developed an understanding of mediation as a form of conflict resolution;
- the ability to present ideas that may be useful in promoting cooperation in early childhood centres in response to posed problems;
- learned how to apply certain strategies in situations in which ethical dilemmas may arise.

BACKGROUND

As this chapter is being written, conflicts in different parts of the world abound and seem more threatening than ever. The peace process, for example in the Middle Eastern countries, seems more precarious and as far away from resolution as it has ever been. Relations between India and Pakistan are highly polarised and the threat of nuclear weapons has escalated conflict, fear and horror. The war against terrorism in Afghanistan has left that country ravaged and destitute. Just what has been achieved through the conflict seen so graphically in war is difficult to imagine given the deaths, maiming, destruction of property and the environment, and the very breakdown of a society. The question must be raised: why is it that in 2002 we seem further away from resolving conflicts constructively than ever before? We must have a better understanding of the theories of conflict, mediation and the importance of sound resolution to conflict, but it seems in many instances that the world is incapable of working towards consensus and achieving it.

It is obvious, then, that managing and achieving a resolution to entrenched conflicts is difficult and requires some cultural changes and acceptances that run very deep. The bringing of conflicts to the negotiating table is in itself a challenge in some instances, and requires mediation by an acceptable, impartial negotiator. Even then, resolution is far from certain as it involves getting people to look beyond their own self-interest.

The nature of conflict

Bolton (1986: 206) says that conflict is unavoidable. To be human is to experience conflict: differences in opinions, values, desires, needs and habits are the 'stuff of daily living'. He goes on to say that 'It is impossible to rise completely above selfishness, betrayals, misrepresentations, anger, and other factors that strain and even break relationships'. He believes that conflict at its best is disruptive and at its worst destructive. As conflict escalates, as it often does, it consumes all the things and the people it touches.

What exactly is conflict: how can it be defined, and what are the elements of it?

Crawley (1992: 10) defines conflict as a manifestation of differences working against one another. This is a very basic yet helpful definition. He proposes that some conflicts can be explosive and cause much damage. This situation has certainly been evident in major international conflicts. Another definition of conflict, by Noone (1996: 3), states that:

> ... conflict arises between two or more individuals, corporations or groups when the fulfilment of the interests, needs or goals of one side is perceived to be

incompatible with the fulfilment of the interests, needs or goals of the other side. Disputes are sometimes based upon truly incompatible, deeply held beliefs and values or fundamentally different world views. However, most of the disputes which go to litigation derive from personal rivalries, domestic incompatibilities and the unending competition for limited social, economic and environmental resources.

Steers and Black (1994: 554) present another useful definition of conflict:

Conflict [is] the process by which individuals or groups react to other entities that have frustrated, or are about to frustrate, their plans, goals, beliefs, or activities. In other words, conflict involves situations in which the expectations or actual goal-directed behaviour of one person or group are blocked—or about to be blocked—by another person or group.

Steers and Black go on to give a number of examples of how conflict can occur, such as when A gets promoted and B doesn't, or when a company finds it necessary to lay off valued employees because of difficult financial conditions. (Both these examples can also be related to working in early childhood situations.)

Crawley differentiates between explosive and constructive conflicts graphically, as in Figure 7.1. The differentiation between explosive and constructive conflict as presented by Crawley gives us a model to consider as we work our way through the issues of workplace conflict.

Conflict may arise in the workplace for many reasons, and it is important to state that some conflict can be constructive and therefore positive in any organisation, including early childhood centres. If conflict generates debates and discussion on important issues then it should be managed effectively to bring about a positive outcome. In most conflict situations leaders will need to assist in managing the conflict, especially if it is related to some potential or actual change. Conflict occurs in the workplace irrespective of the discipline base and in many instances is reliant on the leadership of others to be resolved in a way that is satisfactory to everyone involved.

In addition, Steers and Black (1994: 555) present four different types of conflict:

1. goal conflict—when one person or group desires a different outcome from that which others do;
2. cognitive conflict—where one person or group holds ideas or opinions that are inconsistent with those of others;
3. affective conflict—when one person's or group's feelings or emotions (attitudes) are incompatible with those of others; and
4. behavioural conflict—when one person or group does something or behaves in a certain way that is unacceptable to others.

Figure 7.1 Explosive and constructive conflicts.

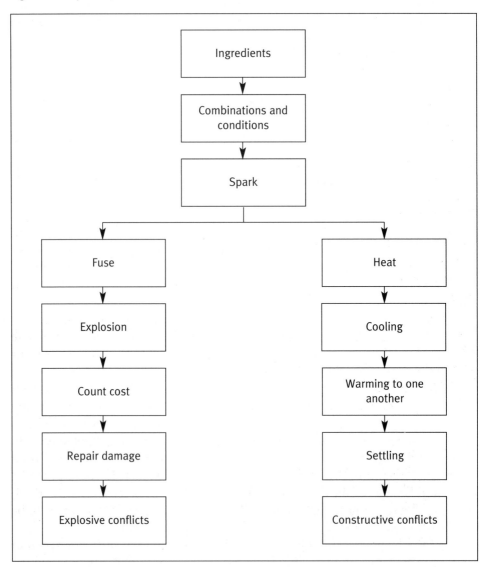

Source: Crawley (1992: 11).

The number of levels of conflict depend on the number of people involved, and one can have conflict limited to one person (a personal, internal conflict) or conflict between any number of organisations.

Conflict is most often viewed in a negative sense, and the feeling is that it has to be eliminated. However, conflict can be either functional or dysfunctional in an organisation. There are situations where conflict can be quite helpful in an organisation—to managers who are attempting to introduce change, for example. Positive conflict can lead to the generation of new ideas or solutions to existing problems, it can stimulate the desire for change and even promote healthy competition between staff members.

On the other hand, conflict can be a negative entity with negative consequences, as when the energies of people are spent in trying to resolve conflict rather than being used positively in the generation of the organisation's product (e.g. good-quality services in early childhood). Negative conflict is one of the main causes of stress in individuals, and where there is a degree of stress among the personnel in an organisation there is also unhappiness, insecurity and diminished productivity.

Bolton (1986: 215) introduced the terms *realistic conflict*, where there are opposing needs, goals and values, and *non-realistic conflict*, which stems from ignorance, error, historical tradition and prejudice, poor organisational structure, displaced hostility, or the need for tension release. Non-realistic conflict can be controlled or prevented using some of the methods summarised later in this chapter.

Before moving on to consider conflict in early childhood settings it is valuable here to look at some of the strategies used in other fields of management to overcome conflict and the negative impact of conflict.

Steers and Black (1994: 564) present five strategies that seldom work and sometimes even exacerbate the problem. They appear to be often-used strategies and are linked to an avoidance approach to resolving conflict situations. These five strategies are:

1.   Non-action—doing nothing and ignoring the problem. The belief here is that if it is ignored it will go away. Often, ignoring a problem only intensifies it.

2.   Administrative orbiting—when managers acknowledge that a problem exists but say that it is 'under study' or 'a committee is looking at it' when in reality little serious action exists.

3.   Due process non-action—when there is an established procedure for redressing grievances but this is a long, costly and tedious procedure, which in the end usually ends up wearing down the people dissatisfied with the cause of the problem.

4.   Secrecy—as when managers attempt to resolve conflict by taking secretive action, as is often the case in pay disputes. It follows the idea that 'what they don't know won't hurt them'. Such an approach leads to a distrust of management.

5.   Character assassination—when the person with a conflict is labelled a 'troublemaker' and attempts are made to discredit this person and distance him/her from others in the group. The belief here is that the isolated person will be 'silenced' by negative group pressure or will leave.

Steers and Black (1994: 566) present a number of strategies for preventing and reducing conflict. For preventing conflict, they offer the following strategies:

- emphasising organisation-wide goals and effectiveness—where the emphasising of the larger goals of an organisation will help employees to see the 'big picture' and, perhaps, work together towards these goals;
- providing stable, well-structured tasks—where the presenting of clear and well-defined work activities that are understood and accepted by employees minimises ambiguity;
- facilitating intergroup communication—where improving the dialogue among groups and sharing information assist in eliminating conflict; and
- avoiding win–lose situations—where resources are scarce, for example, and management introduces some form of resource sharing to overcome possible conflict.

Steers and Black (1994: 567) introduce a number of strategies for reducing conflict, some of which are:

- physical separation;
- the use of rules and regulations;
- limiting intergroup interaction;
- use of integrators (people who 'integrate');
- confrontation and negotiation;
- third-party consultation;
- rotation of members.

A number of these strategies are taken up later in this chapter.

JOB SATISFACTION

There are many issues relating to job satisfaction for staff working in the field of early childhood. Much depends on their training, workplace conditions and the industrial conditions under which they are employed. Teachers, as contrasted with childcare workers, are on very different awards with different salary scales, leave entitlements and daily hours of contact with children and parents. In the main, early childhood services have a majority of female staff, with few male staff. The teaching/caring role is often viewed in the community as something of low value, of poor status and an extension of 'babysitting'. In spite of these factors there are many early childhood staff who get enormous satisfaction from their job, irrespective of the context of their work.

Referring again to Crawley's (1992: 10–11) statement defining conflict, he differentiates between constructive conflict and explosive conflict. Constructive conflict, he says, enables management to:

> ... transform the interaction between the ingredients so that, when the spark occurs, there will be heat generated, but it will not last, destroy the ingredients or damage the surroundings. Rather than exploding, the ingredients will cool, readjust to one another and settle.

Explosive conflicts, he says, contain the following components, which are summarised as:

- ingredients—differences such as age, gender, culture, values, interests, status, role and responsibilities;
- combinations and conditions—the environments in which people live and work;
- the spark—occurs as differences clash;
- the burning fuse—the smouldering of the conflict, that may include behaviours of defensiveness, confusion, jockeying for a position, proliferation of issues and inability to find a resolution; and
- the explosion—a dramatic, violent exchange affecting the people nearby, as well as those involved.

CONFLICT IN EARLY CHILDHOOD SETTINGS

To look at an early childhood discussion on the meaning of conflict we turn to Clyde and Rodd (1989, in Rodd 1998: 62), who propose that:

> Conflict in early childhood settings is a form of interpersonal interaction in which two or more people struggle or compete over claims to beliefs, values, preferences, resources, power, status or any other desire. It is evident that the early childhood context provides a ripe arena for conflicts to emerge given that individual philosophies about caring for and educating young children are derived from subjective beliefs, values and preferences supported by personal experience. In fact, many early childhood staff have reported that dealing with conflict over ethical dilemmas is a major source of tension in the workplace.

What Clyde and Rodd state is unfortunately true, and small teams with bitter differences can mean unhappy workplaces for early childhood staff who have little chance of distancing themselves from disputes. The very nature of their daily work requires staff teamwork at every point if the safety and welfare of children are to be maintained.

Over the past 10 years in many countries, both developed and underdeveloped, we have seen changing policies and practices in early childhood services, many of these for the better (such as the concentration being focused on the care and education of the under-3s in child care). However, early childhood services continue to be vulnerable to the vagaries of funding allocation and government policy changes. In Australia, for example, ongoing changes to Commonwealth government funding have created confusion for centre management and additional work for administrators. Such funding uncertainty has led to fears about centre viability and even job security. Some of these factors have contributed to conflict: if staff or parents are insecure about the viability of a centre, this can affect human relationships and staff interactions.

In recent years, areas within the early childhood field have been subjected to a range of pressures—for example, the rapid expansion in child care in many countries in the early 1990s, where demand outstripped supply. Such rapid expansion sometimes results in staffing crises, with inexperienced, often young staff being employed in positions of responsibility. As a result we have seen the proliferation of some poor-quality programs, particularly in child care. Ways of overcoming these problems are being developed, particularly by governments. A good Australian example of this was the development of a system of accreditation of child care (mentioned in Chapter 2), as quality improvement then became a national issue in Australia as well as in other countries.

Career prospects for staff have presented a problem worldwide for early childhood services. It is only in recent years that some progress has been made towards improving working conditions for early childhood staff and raising their professional standard. However, looking globally, professionalism and career structures are varied, and the status and industrial conditions of these early childhood professionals remain low in most countries in comparison, for example, with other teachers at primary or secondary level.

Some studies consistently show that teaching is a stressful occupation. *The Australian* on 9 June 2002 reported on a recent study in Queensland done by Dr Eva Duggan, who found that the main causes of stress for teachers were:

- student attitudes and behaviour;
- administrators' attitudes and responses;
- parental attitudes and action; and
- time and workload pressures.

The study further led to the comment that 'Externally, it [stress] could manifest as outward, negative expressions, anger, irritability, mood changes, frequent ill health, and the need for "mental health" days'.

A large-scale study of childcare staff in the USA by Phillips, Howes and Whitebrock (1991) showed that while staff were satisfied with their work they were dissatisfied with industrial conditions—salaries, hours of work, and status. Low salary was the main reason given for the high turnover of staff reported.

Given that the definition of early childhood covers the age range of 0–8 years, the range of settings including their physical makeup varies widely. An early-years school setting can, for example, be a class of some 25 children with one teacher in charge. At the other end of the spectrum, a childcare centre catering for young children can have many rooms, with a range of child/staff ratios depending on the ages of the children and the licensing regulations of the state or country. Some centres are purpose-built, others may be house conversions with the necessary structural modifications made in accordance with licensing regulations.

The provision for outdoor play may be generous or, as in some highly industrialised countries like Singapore, children may have no access to the outside environment, provision being made indoors for 'outdoor' activities. What these contexts have in common is that they must be safe for children and that the staff member in charge must have some form of training. Other potential problems include:

- a small amount of space for storage, meetings and staff rooms;
- small areas for greeting parents and children; and
- limited facilities for infants and toddlers.

These features relate to the physical environment, but there are other common work-related problems, including:

- a high level of noise;
- many interruptions, children coming and going, parents coming and going;
- heavy demands on adults' time for attention and care on the part of the children;
- the high level of responsibility placed on teachers and carers for the safety and welfare of children in their care;
- long hours of work, particularly in childcare settings; and
- changes in the program to include specialist teaching for children with disabilities, out-of-school-hours care, play groups, toy libraries, parent groups.

The above are but some of the activities occurring in an early childhood centre. They mean that all staff have to be flexible and able to cope with the many changes happening during a day's work. Whatever the context, early childhood staff are entrusted with great responsibility for caring for a nation's future citizens.

What we are saying here is that the culture of an early childhood centre will vary depending on the context, goals, resources available, and value placed by a particular society on early childhood education and care.

Early childhood centres can be complex places to work in, often requiring staff to work for long hours without a break. Working conditions are a concern especially in child care, where it is difficult to roster breaks and other relief times for staff. If there is a staffing problem—for example, of absenteeism—the staff on duty often have to work overtime without notice. If a parent is late, staff have to wait for a child to be collected. Working in the human services is often quite stressful. Staff go home exhausted after a day of unanticipated changes, emergencies and crises.

Where conflicts arise in early childhood centres they must be resolved quickly. In small centres a staff member often cannot find the space to get away and think things through. Another problem with conflict in early childhood centres is that in order to function effectively there must be good teamwork among staff, which means, of course, that staff rely on each other for the work to be done. Conflict may arise out of many day-to-day functions. It can be related to issues of program management in a centre, behaviour management of children, or be related to work with parents and the community.

We have all had first-hand experience of these difficulties and know how destructive any ensuing conflicts can be. Fortunately, not all conflicts are explosive, but passive conflict (e.g. passive resistance to an agreed change in one element of a centre's work) can be just as damaging and difficult to manage.

Neugebauer and Neugebauer (1998: 236) write that no-one should drive all the conflict out of the life of a centre, but the challenge is to manage dissension so that it contributes to the growth, not deterioration, of the organisation. They state that it is important to encourage healthy conflict, and that conflict among staff is healthy if it:

- generates new ideas, new perspectives;
- provokes an evaluation of organisational structure or centre design;
- brings individuals' reservations and objections out into the open;
- heightens the debate on pending decisions or problems;
- forces a re-examination of current goals, policies or practices;
- focuses attention on problems inhibiting performance at the centre; and
- energises staff—gets them actively involved in the life of the centre.

On the other side of the coin, Neugebauer and Neugebauer (1998: 237) point out the dangers of unhealthy conflict, and the need for intervention when there are signs of it. Unhealthy conflict happens when:

- one person or faction is determined to emerge victorious;
- the focus of the debate changes but the adversaries remain the same;
- discussion never moves from complaints to solutions;
- staff members start taking sides;
- parents or outside parties get drawn into the debate;
- continuing acrimony starts to erode staff morale;
- dissension continues even after a decision is hammered out; and
- debate focuses on personalities, not issues.

One way of preventing destructive conflict is to build effective work teams in early childhood centres; proactive processes will then diminish the likelihood of negative conflict.

Building effective teams is fundamental to early childhood management practice

Due to the nature of early childhood practice, each staff member has to work as a member of a team. If they cannot, perhaps they are in the wrong work-force. Ability to operate as a member of a team is a criterion for employment in early childhood services, particularly when working with the 0–5-year age group. Teamwork often relies on shared decision making. Hayden (1999: 3) writes that 'Shared decision-making is one secret of successful management. The theory behind it is that those who are affected in any way by the outcome of a decision should be involved in making the decision'. This well-tested maxim dates back to early administrative theory. Licensing and accreditation requirements mandate certain child/staff ratios and, apart from family day care, where one adult may care for a specified number of children in a home, this means that a team is necessary when implementing a program.

One of the most important elements of building an effective team is to identify and work towards achieving common goals. In spite of different training backgrounds and qualifications, it is possible for early childhood staff (ideally in concert with parents) to identify and subscribe to an agreed philosophy. A philosophy needs to be achieved through open discussion and identification of what is important and what it is that all staff subscribe to. In working this way, open communication must pervade discussions and time be given to hear the views and problems of all staff. Through negotiation and reflection, an agreed philosophy (including also the goals of the centre) can be identified. A philosophy has to be, of course, compatible with the cultural views and needs of the client group. However, identifying a philosophy is a professional activity of considerable importance. Once the philosophy has been agreed on, staff must work at ascertaining the best way of implementing the philosophy and achieving the stated goals.

Sherry Storm wrote in 1985, and it is still current today, that in any group situation the key to a successful team is the realisation by each member of the group that the common purpose or goal is more important than any one individual's aims. The first priority of the group manager is to reaffirm the commitment to achieving this goal (Storm 1985: 45). If, for example, staff have very different philosophies about how a centre should be managed, then the potential for conflict is great. However, again such differences can be positive if both individuals or groups are prepared to identify the best features of both sides in the debate and come to a common agreement.

In discussing constructive conflict management, Crawley (1992: 132) proposes some helpful ideas for dealing with conflict within groups by focusing on co-working. Co-working is a partnership aimed at utilising the different skills within small teams. This strategy is particularly relevant to the work of early childhood centres, where groups/teams are often quite small in membership.

Likewise, Johnson, LaMontagne, Elgas and Bauer (1998: 3) propose strategies for avoiding conflict. In summary, these strategies are:

- Agree on the basics—that is, identify common goals and how to achieve them.
- Search for interests in common—that is, search for consensus on an issue.
- Experiment—that is, be prepared to try out new, possible solutions.
- Doubt your own infallibility—that is, be prepared to ask, 'Am I sure I am right?'.
- Treat differences as a group responsibility. Conflicts are now to be resolved by the total group.

Neugebauer and Neugebauer (1998: 250) believe that developing a staff of individuals into an effective team can be rewarding, but warn that it is not a quick or painless process. They identify steps in the team-building process as follows. It is necessary to:

- **Set achievable goals.**
  - These should be understood and accepted by all team members.
  - They should be challenging yet achievable.
  - They should be measurable.
- **Clarify roles.**
  - Roles need to be clearly defined and understood by staff.
  - Part of this understanding is delineation of responsibilities.
- **Build supportive relationships.**
  - Some approaches that assist this are to provide training on effective feedback.

- Designate team resource people who have specific skills in certain areas.
- Offer help when needed, still being sensitive to individual needs.
- **Encourage active participation.**
    - Focus on all being encouraged to contribute ideas, opinions and energies.
    - Encourage creative ideas.
    - Show interest in the entire team effort.
- **Monitor team effectiveness.**
    - Evaluate in terms of whether or not the team is achieving its goals.
    - Assess how the team is functioning.

It is proposed that Neugebauer and Neugebauer's approaches are applicable to early childhood centres and could be used as staff development principles in achieving staff cohesion and minimising potential conflict.

STAFF DEVELOPMENT

In many sectors of education large amounts of resources, both physical and human, have been put into staff development in order to bring about needed change and to assist in implementing redirections. This practice is very evident, for example, in departments of education in Australia and some over-seas countries. However, in elements of early childhood, again to mention child care, such resource support has been problematic, as resources have not been made available by governments or systems for staff development. Even in 2002 there are few indicators of any policy changes in relation to support for staff development. Small centres have to work through their management committees (where the service is community-based) or the proprietor (for commercially based centres) to get resources in the form of money and time made available for staff development activities.

An effective staff development program is one of the best ways of raising the professionalism of staff and the quality of programs, both of which are helpful in minimising conflict, whatever form it takes.

Open communication

A vital part of any centre's functioning is the communication that occurs among staff, and among staff and parents and the wider community. Any discussion on conflict resolution in the workplace needs to have a clearly defined position on communication. Conflict can be minimised with open communication when it involves all interested staff. Poor communication may set up barriers, which indirectly contribute to creating conflict. Mohan, McGregor and Strano (1992: 6) make the following suggestions about effective communication:

- Organise the message in terms of its purpose.
- Understand that different channels of communication have different effects.
- Provide receivers with the opportunity to give feedback—that is, an evaluation of communication.

In any conflict situation it is important to find out, by communicating with those involved, exactly what the problem is. One should pose questions that give those involved in the conflict the opportunity to explain clearly what has caused the conflict. Some open questions will allow for sharing of information and perhaps elicit the underlying problems.

Starter questions for an early childhood leader responsible for resolving conflict might include:

- What is the cause of this problem? *Explain why you are angry (or unhappy) about the situation.*
- How can we solve this problem?
- What is the best way to satisfy all parties involved in the dispute? *It is most important to hear all sides of the problem and give everyone an opportunity to discuss it. Sometimes people will be too upset or too distressed to discuss their concern immediately, so sensitive intervention is vital. Timing of discussion is another important factor. Avoid starting at the end of the day, when everyone is tired and wanting to go home.*

Attempting to resolve problems

In attempting to resolve conflict, it is important to:

- be as objective and impartial as possible;
- identify all the relevant information;
- identify quickly what the problem is and in particular what the source of conflict is;
- verify that you have understood clearly all elements of the problem;
- keep all parties focused on the problem rather than on each other's behaviour;
- find a solution that satisfies all parties; and
- be sensitive, but give guidance for coming up with a workable solution.

When resolving any problem, one should make sure that the solution is acceptable and understood by all parties. This can be done by summarising the outcomes of the discussions and presenting the agreed solution.

Sometimes, however, deep-seated differences cannot be solved using the above strategies. What should a person do if it is not possible to resolve conflict in the workplace after many strategies have been attempted? Perhaps mediation is the best option to pursue when direct negotiation between parties has not been effective.

Mediation

The essence of mediation is the commonsense idea that the intervention, through invitation of the parties by an experienced, independent and trusted person, can be expected to help the parties settle their quarrel by negotiating in a collaborative rather than adversarial way (Noone 1996: 5). An expansion of this definition is as follows:

> [mediation is] . . . a process in which an impartial third party called a mediator is invited to facilitate the resolution of a dispute by the self-determined agreement of the disputants. The mediator facilitates communication, promotes understanding, focuses the parties on their interests and uses creative problem-solving techniques to enable the parties to reach their own agreement.   (Noone 1996: 21)

Mediation is not a new approach, although some of the terminology or jargon may be. Noone also explains that societies have traditionally used mediation rather than litigation in an attempt to resolve disputes. In many industrialised Asian countries, mediation is currently the main means of resolution of disputes (Noone 1996: 6).

In looking at the practical application of mediation, Crawley (1992: 187) proposes some ways of getting parties to agree to mediation. These are, in summary:

- Point out the benefits—time and space to express feelings in a neutral setting and a chance to review all the information.
- Point out the dangers of alternative methods—like, for example, litigation, loss of time, work opportunities, continuations and indeed escalation of the conflict.
- Be clear about the role of the mediator—impartiality, ability to control negative behaviour, willingness to listen and to use facilitative communication.
- Be clear about the expectation of both parties—willingness to express feelings, ideas and opinions, and to clarify information.
- Point out the mutual benefit of contact.

Choosing a mediator

Choosing a mediator is a critical element in the total mediation process, as the role requires a skilled professional. Mediators must have no direct involvement in any aspects of the conflict. They must be aware of the confidentiality issues and not divulge any information under any circumstances to outside people. Ideally, in relation to early childhood, they will be in a different field from early childhood in order to be completely impartial.

The actual mediation process

There are many ways of dealing with the mediation process, and students are encouraged to consult the literature widely. However, one of the points worth making here is that mediators sometimes have separate sessions with each party, in order to:

- gather relevant information;
- clarify important issues before bringing the parties together;
- ease any tensions that parties might have about the process; and
- give some opportunity for the parties to ask questions of the mediator, which may lend the whole process more credibility and promote confidence.

First mediation session with both parties

The main purpose of an initial session with both parties is to begin the process and gather initial information, and to get some idea of the depth of feeling of the parties when situated together.

In terms of process, it is important to get an initial statement from each party. How this develops will depend entirely on the context and the intensity of the conflict, and the personal feelings of the parties—in effect, the depth of the conflict. Crawley (1992: 199) writes:

> ... that the mediator acts like a mirror, letting individuals see one another clearly, and on the other hand like a warming rose-tinted spectacles, helping one person to see the humanity of their opponent through the fog of their own hostility. This is the world of 'I'm OK, you're OK' enacted by the mediation process.

Follow-on mediation sessions

After the initial session it is to be hoped that parties will begin talking to one another and confronting the challenging problems. They then move on to identifying some common ground—some agreement as a basis for further negotiation.

In all of the sessions the mediator does not judge or interrupt people in their discussions but tries, in a sensitive way and using skilled questioning, to move them on to identifying common ground. The mediator will strive to get the parties to talk and to listen attentively to one another.

Sometimes mediators construct visual summaries at the end of mediation sessions so that parties can agree on what has been achieved to date. In this, the mediator is drawing attention to any agreement achieved so far and to any issues that cannot be dealt with by mediation and that need resolution in some other arena.

In all, the mediator identifies the progress, emphasising where positive progress has been achieved and providing impartial feedback to the parties. This approach actively moves parties away from conflict and towards cooperation.

Outcome of an agreement as a result of mediation

The ultimate role of any mediator is to lead those in conflict to a point where they can agree to a settlement of their dispute. Here, the mediator needs to make sure that the parties feel that, of their own free will, they have come to an agreement and are satisfied with the outcome. They must feel that they have been empowered in finding a solution to what often seems an insoluble source of conflict. If this process has been really successful the participants should be able to manage conflict situations on their own in the future. This is a measure of the success of the mediation process.

It is important to recognise that, even in contexts where agreement has not been reached, the efforts of people in going through this process are valuable and should be recognised.

The mediation process as outlined is applicable to early childhood contexts and should be considered a viable option when other negotiation processes have broken down, as is illustrated in Case study 7.1.

Case study 7.1

Centre A is located in a busy industrial part of Sydney. This is a centre with 10 staff and a full-time director. Some 300 children attend the centre for a range of programs and for different lengths of time. The staff are very diverse, with a range of qualifications and experience from highly qualified to minimally qualified. The management committee has employed all staff and takes an active role in the management of the centre. The chair of the management committee has asked the director to extend the hours of operation to 11pm as many parents are on

Continued

shiftwork. This request has serious resource implications, both human and physical.

Discussions with staff have reached a stalemate, as no staff are prepared to work beyond 7pm, for personal reasons. The director herself is now in an acrimonious position with the staff, and this situation has been going on for four weeks. The committee has said that the director is in breach of her contract if she cannot resolve the issue, and her employment may be terminated. Staff are now very concerned, as their employment also is threatened.

CAUSES OF CONFLICT IN EARLY CHILDHOOD CONTEXTS

It is useful to consider some of the potential causes of conflict, as being aware of them may help managers to be proactive and defuse situations before they become explosive.

Some of the origins are identified by Rodd (1998: 64), including the following.

- **The physical setting.** Staff often work in small settings in separate rooms, making communication difficult. This situation can be contrasted with other teams working in close proximity in the same centre. Rodd is correct in her views, and we would add that small, sometimes cramped quarters give staff nowhere to escape, even for a short break.

    Rodd perceives communication breakdown in early childhood centres, where the staff have to be closely focused on the children in their care for safety, education and welfare reasons. Such direct focusing sometimes minimises opportunities for good communication with colleagues and team leaders. It is difficult to discuss a problem when staff are not able to give it their undivided attention.

    Rodd also notes that the contact with parents is sometimes problematic. Busy parents 'dropping and collecting' children often do not have the opportunity to experience effective communication with centre staff. Again the physical environment may not be conducive to sharing information fully but communication is rather done 'on the run'.

- **Differing salary scales.** The fact that staff in centres have different qualifications and are employed under different industrial awards is a constant problem for staff. Some staff carry out the same duties as others but their level of remuneration, holiday leave and other industrial conditions are quite different. A person employed under a teachers' award, for example, may be eligible for 10 weeks of holidays whereas a childcare person, employed under a different award, may be eligible for four weeks. The salary gap between a trained teacher and a childcare worker can be in the region of $14000p.a. However, Lyons (1996), conducting a study of staff turnover in childcare centres, found that the most satisfying aspect of the role of respondents was the day-to-day work, not the industrial conditions. This has been found in other studies in the USA (Lyons 1996). While this finding might be true for certain aspects of a childcare worker's workload, it does not deal with the matter of work conditions or the stressful nature of the work—the long hours, low status and poor industrial conditions, including differing salary scales.

- **Complex centres.** The demands of centres offering a wide range of services may make communication and role differentiation difficult.

- **High turnover of staff.** Staff turnover minimises the opportunity to develop a sense of loyalty and commitment. When personnel within a team change often, disruption occurs irrespective of how well managed the process is. New staff have to be inducted and new working relationships formed with children, staff, parents and community members. Complex staff rosters again minimise or complicate meeting times for teams to fully discuss issues and challenges.

- **Staff appraisal.** Difficulties in implementing staff appraisal procedures may occur because some staff find it difficult to accept feedback regarding their workplace effectiveness or ineffectiveness. Appraisal is part of job performance and staff development, and staff who cannot accept this process may find themselves in conflict with their supervisor or centre manager.

- **Emergencies.** Emergencies such as a seriously ill child or a child who has had an accident create stress within the working environment. Staff are working with children who, for many reasons, are highly vulnerable, and the nature of this care and education in times of emergency can create conflicts, particularly regarding priority.

- **Staff development as a team.** Given the long periods of operating time, for example when childcare centres operate for extended hours (including even 24-hour centres), it is difficult to free whole teams to engage in staff development relating to personnel issues, such as managing conflict.

- **Role ambiguity.** The question of responsibility often arises. To whom are the early childhood professionals primarily responsible—the children or the parents or centre management? This question continues to emerge, as in crisis situations parents seek immediate help before being referred to appropriate professionals.

- **The care/education dichotomy.** This is still alive, although sectors of the profession are now working together more closely.

- **Centre policies.** Lack of clarity as to how policies must be implemented can lead to conflict.

- **Code of ethics.** An inability to implement an agreed code of ethics can create ethical dilemmas, which in turn generate unnecessary conflict.

- **Demands made on a centre.** Accreditation reviews or enrolment problems can create concern among staff and, if not managed well, lead to conflict.

- **Career progression.** Lack of, or minimal, career progression opportunities can lead to rivalry among staff.

The early childhood leader as a manager of conflict situations

The effective early childhood leader is well aware of the crucial nature of her/his role in managing and indeed averting conflict in the workplace. However, given the complexity of the early childhood workplace, managing conflict situations is often neither easy nor effective, even trying a range of strategies.

A number of strategies for resolving conflict have previously been mentioned. In addition, the following are helpful:

- Implement an effective system of communication with everyone associated with the centre—children, parents, staff and the wider community.
- With the staff, develop comprehensive policies that are accepted and well understood. Make the effective implementation of all policies a priority.
- Review policies if they are found to be ineffective or to create conflict.
- Clarify the role description and accountabilities of all staff members, both professional and paraprofessional.
- Have an induction program for all new staff members as they assume their duties.
- Conduct staff appraisals at regular, agreed-on intervals and attend to any needed follow-up.
- Try to develop a positive climate of democratic decision making in the

centre. Staff are more likely to accept ideas if they are part of the process.

- Respect the rights of children, staff, parents and the community. Be vigilant about the implementation of this.
- Appoint supervisors who are fair, just and respected by colleagues.
- Be available to listen to complaints or problems before they escalate.
- Encourage teamwork in the centre and make time available for teams to meet to discuss not only program planning but how effective their teamwork really is.
- Make time available to have workshops on what it means to operate within a code of ethics. Working through hypothetical case studies may be helpful. (Workshops may be quite difficult to organise, given the long hours that some centres operate and the shifts that staff have to work. At a practical level, meetings with the whole staff are difficult to arrange and relief staff would have to be employed—again a financial burden.)
- Identify any unusual signs of work stress in staff members. Be proactive in discussing the causes of their stress and identify a solution if the problem is indeed work-related.
- Encourage parents to have realistic expectations of staff in relation to all aspects of a centre's operation, including respecting the rights of staff and valuing their work.

The management of conflict in early childhood services can be complex, but an interview with Jill Huntley, a district coordinator in South Australia, yielded extremely valuable insight into how leaders help others to cope with conflict situations. Ms Huntley has 12 years of experience as a district co-ordinator in different locations and working with a range of diverse services, including preschools, childcare centres, family day care staff, out-of-school-hours care and the first years of school.

Helping early childhood staff to work through conflict situations

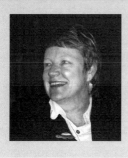

JILL HUNTLEY
District Coordinator
Children's Services
South Australia

Continued

1. What are the elements of leadership that you see as important for encouraging teamwork in early childhood professionals?

The word that immediately comes to mind is 'relationships'. Of prime importance is the establishment of sound relationships based on open communication, trust and confidentiality, which are established and maintained over time. This positive relationship is a two-way process whereby leaders develop sound working relationships with their staff and support them in a variety of ways. They assist staff to develop confidence, grow in their professional role and function as effective team members. Leaders keep up to date and disseminate research findings and information about current trends and developments in the field, both nationally and internationally. They challenge staff to take up new initiatives and give of their best. Leadership takes various forms and will on occasion be an up-front approach and at other times be very subtle and behind the scenes.

2. What are some of the sources of conflict among staff in early childhood centres in your work experience?

The opposite of the relationships statements in the first question—poor relationships, poor communication, lack of information sharing, lack of power sharing and involvement in decision making. All these can cause conflict. If conflict does arise in an early childhood service I attempt to get the conflict resolved as quickly as possible by assisting staff to work through the problem. On occasion I have been a mediator in the process and this has worked well.

3. As a leader, what do you perceive your role to be in these situations?

I see my role as that of a facilitator assisting a team to work through differences and achieve an agreed outcome. If it has been a difficult conflict situation, then I will monitor the situation over time to see that the resolution has been fully achieved.

I see my role as being proactive and upgrading the early childhood profession by helping all service providers understand their work and roles. As well, I assist educators to see that they have common goals with other early childhood services and are not in competition with them but work together to ensure a range of options for families.

There is also a mentoring role for a leader, and this assists in many ways, mentoring new early childhood leaders and supporting staff as they undertake new initiatives—assisting with professional organisations and groups as an advocate in a proactive way. A current example of this is the Future Links Group (birth to 8), whereby seminars have been organised with guest lecturers, newsletters written and disseminated, websites created. As part of Future Links a global café function was organised, and some 90 educators from a range of services came in the evening and participated in lively discussions about provocative questions/statements. All of these types of endeavour build professionalism, upgrade the status of early childhood, and encourage educators to advocate for the early childhood profession in a cohesive and unified way.

Much of our in-service training is in the evening, as it's the only time the

Continued

range of service providers can be free from work commitments and meet. Strong attendance demonstrates commitment and a quest to develop further as professionals: leaders help by engendering such an attitude!

4. How do you help these professionals work through conflict situations?

By strengthening team efforts, by building up trust, by having open discussions about whatever the problem is. By showing staff that as a leader I am interested in the professional development of all team members, not just a leader. By encouraging staff to build support, to network and to be aware of their rights as a person. To remind them of the Early Childhood Code of Ethics. To attempt to depersonalise the conflict situation.

5. In relation to the training of ECE staff, do you see any need to include specific training work on team skills, conflict management etc.?

Training in conflict management is important at both pre-service and in-service levels. People need to know how to manage conflict and to have strategies to use. For example, there are policies against bullying, and no staff in any situation should be subjected to this. Students in training also need work on conflict management as they will on occasion be in less powerful positions.

6. Is there anything else you would like to share about dealing with conflict in early childhood and leadership?

I affirm the importance of leadership, as it is crucial in all elements of professionalism. Assisting others to manage conflict is part of the leader's role.
    Finally, investment for the future, for career development, is vital. Building a strong profession helps all, including families and children.

CHAPTER SUMMARY

This chapter has discussed the management of conflict in the early childhood workplace.

- Conflict is a part of everyday life and in many cultures is violent and entrenched.
- Conflict is seen to be a manifestation of differences working against one another.
- Conflict, as in all professions, occurs in early childhood centres.
- Not all conflict is negative, and it can be positive if it forces the re-examination of goals, policies and everyday practices.
- Positive conflict can generate new ideas and re-energise staff.
- Building effective teams is seen to be fundamental and a proactive way to minimise unhealthy conflict.

- Effective communication is necessary to prevent conflict.
- Familiarity with and acceptance of a code of ethics may minimise conflict.
- The early childhood manager has a responsibility and accountability to effectively manage and, where possible, resolve early childhood conflicts.
- Mediation is seen to be a positive way forward when negotiation breaks down.
- Strategies for dealing with and avoiding conflict are presented.

 Discussion and reflection

1. Consider government changes that have occurred during your time as a working professional. Have these changes been for the better or worse in relation to staff job security?

2. Think of a conflict situation you have experienced or witnessed.

    (a) Was it explosive or constructive?
    (b) Why was this the case?

3. List all of the teaching/caring tasks you might undertake during any one day. Compare these with another colleague.

    (a) How are they the same/different?
    (b) What changes do you have to adapt to in any one working day?
    (c) How many different people do you interact with in any one day?

4. Consider your own early childhood centre. Think of three sources of conflict in your centre.

    (a) Are these still sources of conflict?
    (b) If not, why not?
    (c) How might they be addressed if they are still issues of concern to some staff?

5. Consider the points of Neugebauer and Neugebauer (1998: 236).

    (a) How many of these factors mentioned above could be readily applied to your centre/school?
    (b) Is healthy conflict encouraged? If not, why not?
    (c) Discuss an example of healthy conflict that resulted in a positive outcome for your centre.

6. Again you are asked to consider whether the above happens in your centre in relation to conflict management.

    (a) How does your leader manage such conflicts?
    (b) What positive outcomes have occurred as a result of positive conflict management?

7. Present to a small group the roles of two of the staff you work with.

   (a) How do these members function as a team, and what are the strengths and weaknesses of the current arrangements?
   (b) How much time is allocated to team planning on matters other than program curriculum?

8. Design a staff development session of three hours whereby you will give some tasks to staff on clarification of roles. Plan the overall timetable for this. Plan three task sheets for the team to undertake during the workshop. These should focus on identified aspects of staff development.

9. Comment on the communication processes in your centre. Draw a diagram showing the channels of communication.

   (a) What are the strengths of these?
   (b) How could your system be improved?
   (c) Discuss the communication with non-teaching parties (i.e. the management committee and the community).

10. Think about an instance in your centre where it has been impossible to get consensus.

    (a) Is mediation a way forward with this example?
    (b) Think of a community person not associated with this problem who may act as a mediator. Why would you ask this person?
    (c) What qualities does she/he have that would be useful in the mediation process?
    (d) What would be the consequences of not being able to resolve this conflict through negotiation or mediation?

11. Devise a hypothetical situation in an early childhood centre where mediation is necessary. Role-play through the situation with people taking different roles. For example, first assign a mediator and two disputants. Discuss how the role-play went and then change roles. What have you learned from this exercise?

12. Discuss how the problem outlined in Case study 7.1 could be approached. What are the potential risks and benefits from the view of:

    (a) the management committee?
    (b) the director?
    (c) the staff?

13. Draw a plan of your centre.

    (a) Where do you hold meetings?
    (b) What is the venue like?
    (c) Where do you meet parents?
    (d) How effective is this arrangement?

14. Identify some of the management qualities you would want to see in an early childhood leader.

    (a) How might these qualities assist in preventing conflict in your centre?
    (b) You have just been asked to go on a selection committee for a new director. What three questions will you ask the candidate in relation to conflict management in early childhood education?

15. Plan an induction program for a new staff member that will help this person understand the climate of the centre.

(a) Why have you included the activities on it?
(b) What written material should be given out to new staff, and why?

Chapter 8

Globalisation and the futures

Since the future does not exist, we must all play a part in inventing it . . . the past is gone forever but the future is still ours to determine.   (Robert Burns 1993: vi)

In recent years, globalisation has become the five-syllable terror of political economy. No clove of garlic can keep it at bay; there are no stakes to impale it at the crossroads . . . It distributes its rewards and exacts its tribute with random terminality. The butterfly's wings flutter on one side of our planet, and economic chaos shortly reigns on the other.   (Chris Patten 1998: 210)

A global perspective is the smallest frame within which to view human affairs. Anything less lacks the capacity to deal with the interconnectedness and systemicity that characterise the global system.   (Beare & Slaughter 1994: 52)

This chapter looks at management in early childhood services from a futures perspective. If our understanding of the present encompasses and embraces the concept of a future, then a globalisation perspective must somehow be included in it. Globalisation is not likely to go away. On the contrary, it is likely to strengthen its influence on our world's futures.

As the above quotation of Burns says, the future does not as yet exist. Any consideration of management with a futures perspective has to be speculative, as we do not know what we do not know. There are, however, trends in the present changes that indicate a direction for the future. We must analyse these changes if we are to come up with directions for what might be. If we believe, as the quotation goes 'the future is still ours to determine', it is within our ability to acquire new insight, not only about our everyday practice as administrators, managers and leaders in early childhood services but also about where our practices might/should be heading in the future.

But the above is a tall order, because when writing of leadership and management into the 21st century Nupponen (2000: 9) proposes that tomorrow's leaders and managers will be visionary, building a climate of trust, learning from mistakes, enabling a healthy and empowering environment, flexible, adaptive, decentralised, and creating learning organisations.

Elliott (2000a: 3), in an editorial entitled 'Shaping Early Childhood Futures', states that our vision of what is best for children and families will become increasingly diverse, and governments' quests for ways to curtail cost may conversely result in a 'one-size-fits-all' model which, in fact, decreases service quality. So the challenge to be visionary and yet meet resource constraints of communities and governments is considerable! This is the case in most countries of the world.

 Outcomes

At the conclusion of this chapter, the reader should have:

- developed an understanding of globalisation;
- learnt what the term 'futures' means in relation to early childhood services;
- seen how globalisation and futures are interrelated and how they affect early childhood education;
- formed ideas on how managers of early childhood services might operate in a futures perspective within a global environment.

THE FUTURES AND CHANGE

To some degree the concepts of globalisation and futures, as they relate to where management is heading, are intertwined. It is difficult to separate them. It is also difficult to discuss them without drawing heavily on examples from trade, commerce and industry policies and practices, as management practices in these fields of endeavour influence heavily the management policies and practices of all sectors of public service and hence government. Children's services and education are firmly entrenched in the public service arena.

In Chapter 2 we state that change is one of the certainties of the world. Even tomorrow presents a change from today. Change is often unpredictable, and there will be many surprises as the future unfolds before us. Part of the surprise will be the speed of change, and this speed often outstrips our ability and capability to accommodate it. Books on change and futures written in the 1990s that forecast areas of major change could be said now to be somewhat out of date, as these changes are already with us (e.g. genetic cloning of animal and plant species and the human genome advances).

Beare and Slaughter (1994: 6) state that changes in the next 100 years are likely to outstrip those of the past 1000 years in terms of impact, speed, scope and importance. While some of us might not be around to witness these changes, the children we teach probably will.

It is important that we understand the changes that are going on around us, as they could open up options for the future that we have never before thought of. Change, in the sense of advances in our knowledge and understanding, helps us, if we reflect on it, to reconceptualise the present and have some conception of what the future might be.

In the following, Bettye Caldwell (June 2002) presents her views on possible futures for early childhood.

The futures of early childhood

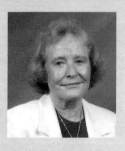

BETTYE CALDWELL
Professor Emerita
University of Arkansas at Little Rock
USA

I am glad the word 'future' was pluralised into 'futures' in the question sent to me, as I don't think the field of early childhood education has a singular future.

Continued

The issues that seem forever to stir up what should be a peaceful and harmonious field are not likely to disappear any time soon. But that is inevitable, in that our field is intimately involved in basic issues of family life, economic stability or uncertainty, and personal and cultural concepts of appropriate social and moral behaviour. We should be proud that the early childhood profession is so intricately interwoven into all those critical aspects of life. However, our involvement does not simplify or lessen our struggle to establish the field along the lines that our own body of knowledge and experience might direct. Rather it seems that, no matter how much we are valued and recognised as a vital service, we invariably are caught up in some of the tumult that surrounds those broader issues.

Recognising that the conflicts in interests and values responsible for creating the tumult are not likely to be resolved any time soon, we can expect continued tension to characterise efforts to increase and improve early childhood services. On the one hand we are lauded as the way to achieve literacy, to solve the welfare-to-work problem, and to allow full development for women as well as men. On the other hand we are occasionally derided as somehow opposed to family values and as distorting, not enriching, the early years for our children. This tension means that the thinkers and innovators whose ideas guide the field can never limit their efforts to the development of proper pedagogy for young children. In addition they always have to show exquisite concern for how that pedagogy will fit into the grid of current and future social conditions and human needs.

Having expressed my conviction that nothing will be particularly easy for us in the future, I will make a few Nostradamus-like predictions:

1. The field of early childhood education (beginning in infancy) will finally achieve status as a legitimate and essential component of lifelong education, and its practitioners will achieve parity with their colleagues in other branches of education in status and compensation.
2. Our programs will be characterised by greater flexibility and more comprehensiveness. The false dichotomy between 'early education' and 'day care' will, due to lifestyle changes, disappear and be replaced by a comprehensive service of educare.
3. Advances in basic research in the areas of brain development and genetic patterning will enable curriculum designers to prescribe teaching/learning practices better adapted to individual differences and thus likely to lead to more efficient learning.
4. The 'early childhood movement' will continue to advance globally and play a major role in the granting of full human rights to women and children—and thus indirectly to men as well.
5. The next century, just as the last, will be a great time to be in the field.

In the introduction to his book *Managing the Future*, Zbar (1994: viii) proposes a number of key features of today's corporate world. These are:

- the globalisation of the market economy;
- the importance of knowledge as the main source of value added; and
- the growing significance of communication and information technology.

These key features he said permeated the writings of the 10 authors summarised in his book. While there were significant differences, he said these three features came through loud and clear from the writing.

Before looking at these features in relation to managing early childhood services it is appropriate to look at what else these authors seemed to agree on. Zbar (1994: viii) said that there was agreement on three significant structural features, namely:

- networks,
- self-employment, and
- teamwork.

Another common thread running through these writers on futures was the philosophy of Total Quality Management (TQM), as espoused by W. Edwards Deming, who elucidated 14 points for management. Total Quality Management is a term used to describe comprehensive efforts to monitor and improve quality within an organisation. The following is a selection of six of Deming's points, as summarised by Zbar for further consideration:

1. Seek to create a constancy of purpose focused on improving both product and service.
2. Stop trying to achieve quality through mass inspection and instead build quality directly into the production process.
3. Train employees on the job.
4. Lead rather than supervise.
5. Break down barriers between the different parts of the organisation.
6. Replace fear with security.

This summary of Zbar's (1994) relates to managing early childhood services with a futures perspective.

GLOBALISATION OF THE MARKET ECONOMY

Perhaps we should define globalisation here. If you look at the introductory quotation of Chris Patten, you might think that globalisation is one of those happenings we could well do without. Simply put, one definition is the opening of markets and the dispersion through technology of market successes (and failures). In one sense globalisation may be a new word but it is not a new concept, as the global migration of people in the 19th century, when people began to move around the world and settle in new places, could be termed an act of globalisation. What we are experiencing today as part of globalisation, in the 'shrinking world' concept or the 'global village' concept, is the ease of ability to transport people, goods, money and information. While people might not be moving as much as they did a century ago, ideas, money and technology—those economic aspects of globalisation—are moving much more rapidly and consistently than ever before and bringing with them those global uncertainties one experiences daily through the vagaries of the stock markets and other monetary indices.

Of course, the condition of world economies affects all countries, and influences the priority the governments of these countries give to funding allocations and to political policies and processes. Decisions on funding across economies have a ripple effect throughout any society, which in turn influences what happens in early childhood services and education at all levels.

The following statement by a Singaporean early childhood educator and proprietor of early childhood services, Julia Gabriel (June 2002), indicates the growing commitment of governments to providing quality services.

Futures for early childhood education

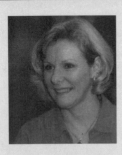

JULIA GABRIEL
Director
Julia Gabriel Centre and Chiltern House Child Care Centre
Singapore

South-East Asia is adapting to increasing numbers of educated, dual-income households. In the past three decades parents have relied on family members to supervise young children at home. Even though this help may still be available, today's parents see increasing pressure facing their children and want them to enter education as early as possible.

Awareness of the importance of early childhood education has led the Singapore government to focus on the content of childcare and preschool programs. This focus will spread to other countries in the region, resulting in overall improvement in quality, particularly through training for early childhood educators. Young girls with minimum levels of education who have traditionally cared for our youngest students will be replaced, over time, with well-trained, conscious providers, speaking high levels of more than one language.

As early childhood educators reconceptualise the future, highlighting the value and importance of the early years, I foresee a continued, corresponding improvement in the focus of governments, parents and educators. Programs for infants and toddlers, involving parents, will become more common. Early childhood

Continued

centres will become more professional and nurturing, and be held accountable for outcomes. Teachers will work in collaborative partnership with parents and students. Communication and understanding will improve.

The cost of early childhood education will rise correspondingly. High quality, particularly in teacher training, comes at a cost. As families become smaller, a trend in North and South-East Asia, parents are more willing, and able, to pay for the best for their children. Such intense focus by parents on their children brings with it high expectations. Whether these high expectations are realised, and at what cost to the child and the profession, is unclear. I foresee a rise in private early childhood education, with centres developing unique personalities and specialisations. The end result: a healthy rise in quality, vitality and choice of early childhood facilities.

Globalisation and early childhood centres

Ideas now flow at an ever-quickening pace, and this aspect is important in our consideration of the effects of globalisation on our early childhood services. You just have to look at the current ideas shaping curricula, caring and teaching methods, materials, equipment, technologies and so on to see that these ideas are worldwide. For example, it is interesting to see how 'constructivism' as it relates to teaching/learning methods is currently influencing early childhood thinking in many countries.

International conferences, visiting academics and practitioners from all over the world influence the policies and practices of governments and systems. Organisations such as UNESCO, the World Bank, UNICEF and others with a global influence also are part of both the global market economy and the global education and care communities.

Sue Harper (May 2002) has made some comments on changing practices from the perspective of a former chief executive director of a childcare centre.

Globalisation

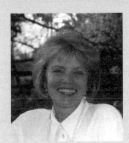

SUE HARPER
President, l'Organisation Mondiale pour l'Education
Préscolaire (OMEP) Australia, and
former chief executive director, Lady Gowrie Child
Centre
Melbourne

Continued

I often wonder what the future will bring. More than ever before, the shape and form of our lives are difficult to predict, as change has been so rapid. At the beginning of the past decade it would have been hard to imagine the speed of the change that has occurred.

When I took up my position at the Lady Gowrie Child Centre in November 1990 there was one computer and one facsimile machine. The computer rested on the desk of the bookkeeper and each week she entered figures according to calculations that had been made manually using a calculator, a pencil and an eraser. In the space of the next 10 years the environment altered, and many computers now provide the machinery to pay salaries, levy fees, maintain databases, manage a training program and design catalogues and brochures. Mobile telephones, computers and the Internet have all had a major impact on our lives.

Coupled with this technological change there have been societal changes. Family structures and relationships, work patterns and career options have all shaped current daily lives.

What do these rapid changes mean for early childhood programs? Do playrooms reflect contemporary society? Consider the home corner—conventional stove, no microwave, an iron and ironing board, a clothesline, the telephone. Is there a computer in the playroom, I wonder?

Do the hours of operation meet the needs of the local community? How do you resolve the tension that exists between parental needs and children's needs? What are the implications for the developmental needs of children?

Children's services are well placed as access points to plan programs that will help and support children to become capable, competent, flexible and resilient. The environment must be relevant, accepting and meaningful for both parents and children; and the services provided must be adapted to meet the individual needs of specific communities. These factors have implications for the location of buildings and the use of multidisciplinary teams of staff and resource people so as to build capable, competent, flexible and resilient communities.

The underlying need for humans is a sense of belonging to families, groups and communities.

KNOWLEDGE AS THE MAIN SOURCE OF VALUE ADDED

Charles Handy, one of the authors in Zbar's book, wrote *The Age of Unreason* in 1932. He described one kind of organisation as 'the Triple I organisation', which encompasses intelligence, information and ideas. These three 'Is' are today's sources of 'value-added'. As summarised by Zbar (1994:115), the people in the 'Triple I' organisation are paid to think and do, and management is based on persuasion and consent rather than on command. Individual and group work is supported by the use of smart machines such as personal computers and robots. Each of the members of the professional core will not only possess their own area of expertise but will also have to be a manager. In the course of their work everyone will be involved in managing projects, people and money. (It could be argued that the people currently engaged in managing early childhood services see themselves as being quite some distance from 'Triple I' management practices, inasmuch as they have little support of 'smart machines and robots' but are slaves to the minutiae of management.)

Handy's 'age of unreason' is characterised by discontinuity (change is faster and less predictable); small things (often the smallest changes will have the most impact); infotech and biotech (technology, economics and biotechnology); and thinking upside down (thinking that challenges the existing order of things, new and different ways of looking at old and familiar problems). An organisation is facing discontinuous change when its past does not prepare it for the future (Limerick & Cunningham, in Zbar 1994: 64).

The following statement by Pam Winter (May 2002) discusses knowledge as being 'value-added', and holds that in relation to the futures we have to take some leadership from the children themselves.

Leadership from children

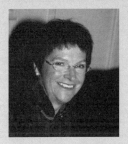

PAM WINTER
Curriculum Policy Officer, Birth–3 years
Department of Education, Training and Employment
Adelaide

In response to the questions: What do you believe the futures for early childhood education might be? What changes can we expect to see as early childhood educators reconceptualise the futures for early childhood? I make the following observations.

How can anyone hazard a guess as to what the future might be? If we were certain about anything it would stop us seeing other ways of doing things. Living with ambiguity and doubt are going to be our assets, for if we do not live with them we have no reason to reflect on how things are and consider alternatives — alternative ways of perceiving, understanding and behaving.

We'll need to consider that there are multiple perspectives to most things and be able to question underlying assumptions and not take things at face value,

Continued

remembering that all understandings are influenced by time and place. The bene-fits of working and learning together for richer understandings will be important. Critical reflection, open-mindedness, flexibility, capacity to form, express and debate an opinion and show deep respect for others are the dispositions that I think will be our strengths. The capacity to gather, sift and critique information and then construct understandings is becoming increasingly valuable. Disposi-tions such as these are learned by children in environments in which they are modelled and practised.

In addition, an ethical framework will help, so that we can think deeply and critically about the options that technology is making possible. There is so much in the world that requires a commitment to interdependence for a more just society and for the sustainability of both our physical and social global environ-ments. We won't survive as a society if living in harmony and rejecting violence don't become our collective priorities. Our children as well as our adults must become more politically and socially aware of what is happening around us and share the responsibility for bringing about changes.

Children, in their early childhood years, are capable of understanding that there are alternatives to almost everything, and it is our responsibility as educators to foster in children of all ages the capacity to think critically, to reflect on their actions and the actions of others, so that they will themselves grow in an understanding of their world and all that is in it and be positioned to make a contribution.

This all sounds very heavy. I think there will always be a need for fun, and time to enjoy friendships and each other's company, time and space to escape, some fantasy, and ways and opportunities of expressing ourselves creatively. Most of all, we will need each other.

Looking at this key feature from the early childhood management perspective we can see clearly enough the importance of 'intelligence, information and ideas'. The old saying that 'information is power' is correct in management. Ideally, managers act on sound information. The early childhood manager has to be knowledgeable of what is happening and what is 'likely' to happen. To be clairvoyant, hardly, but alert to possibilities, yes. To have ideas, yes, and to challenge the status quo, always! However, in challenging anything, particu-larly the status quo, the good manager has to have her/his facts right at the beginning and to have a clearly thought through alternative for consideration. The influence of what is called 'infotech' is increasing in early childhood centres as more of our young children become confident users of the communication and information technologies. It is important that the staff in the centres themselves become confident users. Staff who are 'one page a day' or 'one step ahead of the children' are hardly likely to enthuse and extend the children's knowledge and skills.

By contrast, the South Australian Curriculum Standards and Accountabil-ity Framework (SACSA) of 2001 mentioned in Chapter 2 noted that:

> *As people are exposed to globalisation cultures through the media, consumer products and information technologies so traditional structures are being challenged. The interaction of diverse cultures, both locally and globally, impact on individual and group identities. It is almost impossible to be isolated from the products, images and messages that circulate around the globe and merge with established traditions and practices to shape new meanings and cultures.*
>
> *In children's services and schools we recognise the implications of these increasingly fluid social relations, including the diversity of learners and their wide-ranging and new needs in curriculum and teaching practices.   (SACSA 2001: 5–6 in Department of Education Training and Employment 2001)*

As has been mentioned in Chapters 2 and 5, the SACSA Framework is very innovative. Indeed, it is futures-oriented. Within the Framework five essential learnings have been identified: futures, identity, interdependence, thinking, and communication. Of particular relevance to this chapter is the essential learning 'futures'.

SACSA (2001: 13) outlines 'futures' as follows:

> *What knowledge, skills and dispositions are required to maximise opportunities in creating preferred futures?*
>
> *Learners develop a sense of optimism about their ability to actively contribute to shaping preferred futures and capabilities to critically reflect on, and take action in, shaping preferred futures.*
>
> *Curriculum developed from this Framework provides opportunities and skills for learners to critically examine future possibilities and challenge commonly held assumptions about the past, present and future. Through such analysis learners understand that the future has connections with the present and the past, and that social, political economic and physical environments are constantly changing and can be improved. Thus the major theme of this learning is creating sustainable natural environments, and just and sustainable human environments.   (SACSA 2001: 13 in Department of Education Training and Employment 2001)*

THE GROWING SIGNIFICANCE OF COMMUNICATION AND INFORMATION TECHNOLOGY

This key feature of today's corporate world has already been introduced. Schools, within the present context of compulsive technological dynamism, competition, individualism and radical loss of meaning and purpose, are put in an impossible situation. They stand at the crucial interface between past and future—with the conservation of the culture and with its radical renewal (Beare & Slaughter 1994: 15). While there is an element of truth in what is said by Beare and Slaughter, especially the comment about compulsive technological dynamism and a growing trend towards competition even between schools in the public arena, the comment on radical loss of meaning and purpose is questionable.

What is important, getting back to Zbar's key feature, is that communication is becoming more significant to the success of management in caring and educational establishments. Parents and the community want to be informed of what is happening in their early childhood centres and schools, and it is their right that this information be passed on. Such action makes for a not-too-subtle change in the shift of power and influence in care and education circles. As a result, early childhood and school managers have been forced to change their way of viewing their responsibilities and their practices. Communicating and reporting practices have changed and, one hopes, become more meaningful as a result.

Zbar (1994: viii) went on to state three significant structural features that came from the authors on futures management included in his book, namely networks, self-employment, and teamwork. In relation to managing early childhood services, these features are important and relevant.

Networking in management implies the move from isolated production units to networks of units where collaboration, partnership and alliances are the order of the day (Limerick & Cunningham, in Zbar 1994: 61). We see this movement clearly in early childhood as many independent early childhood centres—mainly childcare centres in Australia, but in other countries this would include preschools as well—form an alliance with others, thereby creating a consortium of one kind or other. For example, many proprietors of commercial childcare centres have a number of semi-independent centres operating within the ambit of the larger, umbrella organisation. There is in such organisations the pursuit of a common goal, with the managers of the semi-independent components collaborating for the greater good of the larger organisation. This practice is a form of networking.

According to Limerick and Cunningham (Zbar 1994: 66), networking is not without its problems, such as:

- inadequately defined purpose and lack of clarity about network boundaries;
- the desire for unit sovereignty at the expense of the network;
- asymmetry between partners (the lack of equality);
- excessive concentration on the short- rather than the long-term goal; and
- difficulties inherent in managing across different cultures.

It is difficult to say whether any or all of the above-named problems are current in any consortium or network of providers, as there are many variations of networks. It is, however, important for us to recognise that such problems could exist.

Self-employment and *teamwork*, as the terms imply, are part of small operations. Many establishments in early childhood services are managed by self-employed people who also employ a small team of workers in accordance with their centre's operation, size and licensing requirements. In the better-run centres the quality of the staff teamwork is often what contributes to the success of the operation.

Another useful perspective on early childhood futures is that of Leah Adams (August 2002). Professor Adams forecasts a future need for multicultural understanding and appreciation of others, not only in a global sense but in neighbourhoods as well.

The futures of the early years

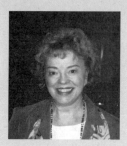

LEAH ADAMS
Professor Emerita
Eastern Michigan University
USA

I believe that in the future early childhood education will recognise, ever more strongly, the importance of the early years in development of the individual. Not only will there be attention to development of the brain, but more attention will be given to the social and emotional aspects of overall development. Our mental alertness, mental stability, emotional capacity, and emotional control will be recognised as being of great importance as the world community continues to struggle for global understanding, tolerance and peaceful coexistence.

In the future, the world will need creative, innovative thinkers, and compassionate, caring people who are healthy both physically and mentally. The need for multicultural understanding and the appreciation of others will intensify, not only in a global sense but also in each and every neighbourhood. Early childhood professionals must continue to look at what can be done in the early years for cognitive growth, also for mental and physical health and the beginnings of working positively with others.

In this chapter we have had the benefit of four statements of significance about the futures of early childhood. In the main these statements have been optimistic and stress the need for us to be futures-oriented in our thrust. Elliott (2000b: 6) writes that 'the future of the world lies with our children, but they need us to make that future safe, peaceful and caring'. Elliott further says that these visions for children send a strong message to early childhood educators. Only through getting together and building thoughtful programs, and through staying in touch with our own childhood, can we help children discover a world full of hope, promise and peace.

Consider now, briefly, and from a futures perspective, some of Deming's management points mentioned on page 215.

MANAGEMENT POINTS

Constancy of purpose and focus on quality

There is no question that quality in early childhood services is very much on the minds of everyone concerned with the care and education of young children. And research reports, such as the recent Australian study by Margetts (2002) in Melbourne which questioned the effects of long-term child care on children's later adjustment to schooling, highlight this continuing concern. Government policies and funding strictures, political action by women, particularly working women, and many other factors are keeping early childhood education and care in the current public arena. Quality, as a topic, has already been introduced in this book (see Chapter 2). Put in a futures perspective, quality, however shown and proven, will be the measure of the survival of early childhood services. Parents, the public and governments are becoming ever more conscious of the importance of quality services for young children's development.

Achieve quality by building it directly into the processes

While this point may be more appropriate to manufacturing production industries, it does apply also to the human service provisions such as early childhood care and education. The Australian Quality Improvement and Accreditation System is one strategy (introduced in Chapters 2 and 4) whereby quality and subsequent practices that reflect quality can be built into the 'system'. Again, from a futures perspective, quality is the yardstick for success in the early education and care 'enterprise'.

Train employees on the job

In relation to early childhood services, in most countries of the developed world licensing regulations set by governmental authorities require a certain level of training for all employees. Implied in this point is that there should be continuous training during employment in the form of in-service training and development. Through such practice an organisation, and hence an industry, can keep abreast of new developments, trends, and the needs of 'consumers'. From a futures perspective, in-service training of an organised kind might become mandatory for continuing licensing.

Lead rather than supervise

Leadership has also been discussed in Chapters 1 and 2. The point being made here relates directly to the value of leadership over supervision. The emerging role of senior management in our customer-driven organisations (including early childhood organisations) is rapidly becoming one of leadership—setting the directions for the organisation, no matter what its size. The leader has to communicate a vision throughout the organisation, taking into account the predictability and unpredictability of the environments in which the organisation operates. It is this latter point that is becoming more prevalent in leadership. Steers and Black (1994: 380), discussing the need for managers to behave rationally, said that if managers choose to ignore an unpredictable environment and consider it to be stable, the end result might not be a high degree of organisational success in the long term. If managers know the environment is unpredictable but ignore it, the same could happen. The accurate perception of good management coupled with high rationality leads to effectiveness.

From a futures perspective for early childhood services there is a degree of both predictability and unpredictability—the former, inasmuch as there will always be a need for children's services (child care and preschooling) as societies have come to embrace such services and expect them; the latter, inasmuch as the external environmental factors of the economy, government and politics, natural resources, technology and demographic changes all will influence possible futures because they influence the sources of demand for services.

Break down barriers between different parts of the service

Certainly the barriers that have previously existed between childcare services and preschooling have been broken down to a degree, but there are still barriers there. A good example of such a barrier is the condition of employment of personnel in both services—differences in salaries, hours of employment, leave entitlements, award salaries and so on. It is not surprising therefore that a prevailing perception exists that as a service profession, child care is inferior to preschooling. There is still a way to go, in the minds of people using the service, the policy makers and governments, and the trade union people to counter this perception. From a futures perspective, the movement already begun to break down remaining barriers has to be intensified. Concentration on training and qualifications, salaries and conditions of service will help speed up the inevitable change.

Replace fear with security

From a futures perspective, this point for management could be the hardest to achieve in the short term in early childhood services. The problem is certainly linked to the environmental predicability and unpredictability mentioned above as well as to conditions of service, status, salary and people's perceptions. It is a psychological truism that people who feel secure—who are secure in their workplace and feel valued—perform better, are better employees and have superior output (in the case of early childhood, the quality of the services provided) to those who fear for their existence. Feeling secure is as much a state of mind as it is a fact of employment. There are many employees in the various workforces who are insecure simply because they themselves know that they cannot do the job expected of them. Here, the matter of staff development is important for management consideration.

In summary, so far we have tried to show that the world of early childhood and the services provided to support parents, families and children are in a constant state of flux, including instability, and that there is nothing to indicate that in the short-term and long-term futures this state of change is likely to disappear. Managers in early childhood services have to work within and around the factors of stability and instability, ignoring neither if they are to remain 'on top' and if their organisations, no matter how small, are to remain viable in the future. We are talking here about managers being in a state of continuous adaptation for survival.

Noam Chomsky (1996: 70) spoke of goals and visions, where vision is a conception of the future and a future society that animates what we actually do. Goals are the choices and tasks that are within reach, that we will pursue one way or another, guided by a vision that may be distant or hazy. The early childhood services manager must have a vision—one that rests on a concept of human nature, of what is good for young people who will be the adults of tomorrow, of their needs and rights, of aspects of their nature that should be nurtured, encouraged and permitted to flourish for their benefit and that of others. This, for early childhood, is advocacy, of what the future might be for children, families, and the purpose and style of early childhood services.

Let us now look more specifically at early childhood services and preschools and schools as they view the future in an uncertain world.

MANAGING THE FUTURES IN EARLY CHILDHOOD SERVICES

In a foreword to the book *Education for the Twenty-First Century* by Hedley Beare and Richard Slaughter (1994), Barry Jones makes an interesting observation. He says, in effect, that our schools are being shaken by their roots because we are paying the price now for our failure to confront global, long-term issues in a time of technological revolution.

Is our education system capable of bearing the weight we will need to place on it? A century ago, schools would probably have provided about 40 per cent of all the information about the world that young people received, reinforced by contact, in and out of class, with their peer group. Home and church/Sunday school would have had more collective input than books or newspapers:

> *Schools once set the information agenda, although that term was not used, while home and church set the moral agenda. Now the cultural agenda is set electronically. Schools and even homes seem to have become part of the counter-culture, the resistance, fighting back with a declining share of the action.   (Jones, in Beare & Slaughter 1994: ix)*

The fundamental assumptions we have about early childhood preschools and schools have to be revised. It is not, as many people would believe (including our politicians), that it should be more of the same, adding a year to compulsory schooling, making it necessary in most cases for formal schooling to begin at age 4 years. Some countries begin the 'formality' of schooling at an even earlier age. Something more radical has to happen to what goes on in those years of preschooling and schooling if there is to be any real change in the capacities of young people to manage their futures.

Certainly schools and school systems are trying to change in ways that will better accommodate what the futures might be, and there have been some successes. People working in the early childhood years could say that the degrees of change to meet the unknown requirements of the future are not so great in early childhood education as they might be in later childhood. Birth is birth and the early years need the nurturing and developmental stimulation that has been the 'content' of early care and education for a long time. Such a view is singularly short-sighted, as not only is development a continuous process but there is sufficient evidence in our knowledge of human development for us to know that children are capable of achieving more than we have previously given them credit for.

In relation to our somewhat static, preconceived ideas of human development, capacities and capabilities to adapt to change, Beare and Slaughter (1994: 7) state:

> *We are, in other words, at a major historical divide . . . This transition away from what we have taken for granted affects the viability of all institutions and the life*

of every individual. Yet, curiously, there is little evidence that those who are running schools and school systems are aware of the implications of these rapid, fundamental and structural changes. In fact, the futures-related tools and techniques which have been developed and applied in other contexts for more than forty years are simply not part of the standard equipment of teachers or of school administration, of educational policy-making or of parent participation in their children's education.

Another viewpoint on the magnitude of change was presented to the 'Revolution 97' conference in Adelaide some years ago and reported in *The Advertiser* (date unknown). The newspaper reported Professor John Tiffin of New Zealand as saying:

The changes [in education and schooling] are going to be much faster than we imagined only two years ago . . . students would be able to travel to their 'virtual school' without leaving home. The schools that existed in cyberspace, required no buildings, carparks or other infrastructure . . . Virtual reality goggles and gloves, voice recognition technology and a force-feedback datasuit could combine with powerful computer systems to enable students to see, talk to, feel and manipulate their virtual environment . . . They would be able to chat with friends from around the world . . .

and so the report went on. It is difficult for our minds to take in the meaning of all the above comments and how they might influence the early childhood years. One thing is for sure: the changes indicated here will influence what early childhood teachers do. In the newspaper report, Professor Tiffin also advised that at that time Spain had a virtual university operating. How long before there will be a virtual primary school? Is it conceivable that there could be a virtual kindergarten?

Beare and Slaughter (1994: 19) present what they see to be a consensus of several aspects of a new world view.

First, the industrialised culture of yesteryear will change dramatically the way we view society, work, wealth, living patterns and the nation-state. These changes imply change in employment patterns—a change already beginning in a dramatic way. The economic uncertainties that seem now to be a part of everyday life affect family life and how people relate to one another and so on.

Second, the condition of the planet and of its delicately balanced ecology is forcing people everywhere to think globally and see themselves differently in the world. The 'greenhouse effect' is now common knowledge, and is causing the global warming that we all are experiencing. The 'business as usual' attitude is no longer acceptable where the world's ecological future is concerned. The authors comment that parents, politicians, public and educators need to adopt quickly this global 'new world' view and way of thinking about the world and to construct with the rising generation a different frame of thinking, both about the world and their place in it. Herein lies the importance of such viewing, thinking and acting in early childhood education.

Third, educators have gone beyond scientific materialism and confidence in the scientific method as the one best way to knowledge, and have embraced other integrative ways incorporating empirical, rational and spiritual dimensions. The authors explain that, as social patterns change, the configurations of towns and cities change, occupational patterns change, education changes, and everyone is affected somehow and to differing degrees. Arguing against the scientific method that is central to subjects, the parts/whole idea, they say:

> *For the 21st century we had better discover quickly how schools in particular can sponsor a different orientation: in place of fragmentation, wholeness and connectedness; in place of devastation and disease, health and balance.   (Beare & Slaughter 1994: 61).*

The managers of early childhood services have a huge task ahead of them if they are to embrace what this new world view implies. The simple facts that many of the world's children exist in poverty, that malnutrition is rampant in over half the world's population, that AIDS and other terminal illnesses are on the increase and affect childhood in ways that the other half of the world cannot understand, are part and parcel of the early childhood educator's knowledge and attitude base. Helping young children to become aware that what they have is a blessing and to use it wisely and accommodate it into their futures is probably an impossible task but one that has to be attempted. It is the task of educators of children of all ages to build perspectives about the future in everything they do.

Burton and Dukes (1990: 163) put the implications inherent in the above paragraph succinctly:

> *Social interventionist programs in the human services can, by themselves, do little to overcome the problems of today in society. There is, however, a growing appreciation of the source of social problems. There is an accumulation of people who have been neglected and catching up is impossible without a major shift in priorities especially in the developed, industrial countries. Social problems that arise out of class and ethnicity are likely to overwhelm many societies.*

Empowerment

Good managers empower people. Good teachers empower their children. Empowerment means looking ahead positively—it is futures-oriented. The opposite of empowerment, disempowerment, also implies a state of helplessness. Young children and young people in general are positive thinkers and movers until such time as this positive trait has been forced out of them in some way by society and society's instruments (the media, schools perhaps, political oppression). It has been said, as a result of surveys of children's thinking of the future, that they are fearful of the future. Much of what they are fearful about comes from other people and the media, more so than their own considered opinions, especially at a young age. These are times when the teachers of these young children can be positive, showing the children how they can take their place in their society and do things to make it a better place now and in the future. This is empowerment. This is the role of the early childhood teacher. It is the role also of the parents, the church and other organisations that have an influence on the children's development and outlook.

When we empower people we give them the capacity to confront not only the present but also the future. (Children who are disempowered, for one reason or other, do not try even to confront the now, let alone an unknown future. They are today's failures, and it is terrible to be a failure at age 5, 6 or 7 years.) It is this feeling of optimism that is important for both children and their teachers in everything they do. An optimistic person of any age will have a go at doing most things and will not give up at the first sign of failure. What you have learnt about the way children learn is important here, as you know that children are not just passive recipients of facts and figures but are active participants in their learning. They construct their world from the many experiences they have from the situations adults and teachers present to them.

Empowered people operate as much in the future tense as they do in the present. Their motivation to be successful has more to do with the future than it has with the past. Success generally brings with it a change in a person's attitude, as they see that they can do things and be someone. Success also brings with it a new understanding of choice, that there may be several ways of doing things and that choice in decision making is possible. We are talking here about a futures perspective to learning and developing. It is up to teachers also to have this perspective and to capitalise on it with their students, no matter what their age. It is a concept of the future—a positive concept, not an abstract, intangible thing.

The empowerment model for teaching and learning may appear to go against the current model used in educational circles, where facts and information are acquired only to be used at examination time or when called on to be used in tasks or projects set by teachers. This approach is more past-oriented than futures-oriented, and has little of the creative process in it. A futures approach—the delving into the unknown, the what might be—is a creative approach, often with limitless possibilities for outcomes.

Beare and Slaughter (1994:105) devote their thoughts to education as empowerment and the futures, saying that:

> ... futures in education is most centrally concerned with negotiating and exploring new and renewed understandings about our present cultural transitions

beyond the industrial era. It has a role to play in defining and creating a more just, peaceful and sustainable world. Visions and views of desirable outcomes always come before their realisation.

Also:

. . . without the future or futures there would be no plans, purposes, goals, intentions, meanings . . . or curricula . . . It is characteristic of our species that, while the body may be time-bound through biological necessity, the mind and imagination are not. An empowered person, adult, teacher, child is futures-oriented.

Early childhood professionals would to be more oriented to empowerment in their methods of interacting with and teaching their young children than their counterparts working with older children and youth. This may be true, but there is always the need for teachers at all levels to reflect on their methods of teaching and the nature, interests and motivations of their children. There are many stresses and strains on teachers of all educational levels, the early childhood level included. How teachers cope with these stresses and strains and how they sieve them is important so that these are not reflected in what they do with their children. If children in learning situations are placed under stress they will not perform as well as if the stress were not there. (There is a difference between stress and being encouraged to learn.) Stress results in conformity, and conformity is related to the here and now. It is related also to disempowerment more than to empowerment. The ideal situation is where both the teacher and her/his children are empowered—to be and become.

GLOBALISATION

The quotation by Chris Patten (1998) at the beginning of this chapter clearly contains the implication that globalisation is here to stay and that it casts its influence over everything that is done, in all walks of life, throughout the world. Globalisation is inherent in all we have said so far, even if it has not been mentioned specifically, as there is always a global agenda to any consideration of futures.

Chris Patten was the last British Governor of Hong Kong. He led the then colony to its reunification with China. His book *East and West* (1998) provides interesting reading on the subject of globalisation, not only because it covers the history of globalisation through human movement over the centuries but because it considers the current economic and educational implications of globalisation. Patten considers, as an educated observer, the educational outputs of Asian countries and those of Europe and the USA. The current emphasis placed on education by Asian countries produces results but, according to Patten, at a price, whereas in the Western countries there is a perceived educational complacency. He does make the following observation, relevant here:

> Yet another of the uncelebrated, or at least undercelebrated, boons of globalisation is to shine a spotlight on the importance of education in a world where jobs, ideas, information and knowledge will travel ever faster and (we should ensure) with fewer and fewer restrictions. And if, in Western societies, governments give their citizens a little more room to breathe, ending the public monopoly of welfare and limiting what they themselves do to what they need to do and can do best, perhaps we can ourselves rediscover a few remaining deposits of community adrenalin, a zest and enthusiasm that will help us to tackle more effectively the social and economic problems of fatigued success.   (Patten 1998: 242)

It is not appropriate in this chapter to go into global matters of economics, trade, politics, concepts of 'the free world' versus whatever the other may be called, ideas that 'you are either with us or against us' and so on. These and many other matters affecting the global world are worthy of study by everyone at an appropriate age and time. As teachers working with children in their early childhood years, we have to be able to appreciate what can be introduced and how it can be introduced and developed. For example, the matter of global warming is one that everyone must be concerned about, as already the effects of the earth's warming are being felt everywhere by countries, societies, families and, hence, children. Chomsky (1994: 188) has the following to say about global warming, and from what is written here it can easily be seen as a topic appropriate for young children's understanding:

> There was a study that came out in Science magazine about a month ago reviewing recent studies on global warming. The possibilities they were considering as plausible were that if the year 2000 goals on carbon dioxide emission are met, which is not likely, then within a couple of centuries, by 2300, the world's temperature would have increased by about ten degrees Centigrade, which would mean a rise in sea level that would probably wipe out a good bit of human civilisation as it's currently constituted. Of course this doesn't mean that the effects set in in three hundred years. They start setting in much sooner . . . The same study says that in order to avoid this it will be necessary to undertake quite radical changes of a kind not even contemplated.

Our goal, as teachers, with children at all ages is to help them to see what they are doing and what they want to do from a futures perspective and to see these things, where appropriate, from a global perspective. Simple messages and activities, such as being concerned about the proliferation of litter in streets and parks and rivers, have a global and futures perspective, and the effective teacher takes the children's thinking beyond the here and now to the 'what might be'.

There is no simple recipe for globalisation in early childhood thinking and action. A global, futures orientation is something that is built up over time. However, it has to start somewhere, and the early childhood formative years are as good a time as any to inculcate in children that sense of responsibility and understanding of outcomes that are the basis of effective citizenship.

A teacher's global agenda, according to Beare and Slaughter (1994: 119), consists of:

- how to clear up the existing mess (the links between our wellbeing and that of the environment, e.g. water pollution);
- how to make the shift towards sustainable economies (many problems of past practices and the nature/human interactions of the past, e.g. farming practices and industrial waste);
- deciding what we want to achieve with our innate capacities, with our technologies and with the earth (conflict between our present 'good life' and what we should be doing with what we have); and
- exercising foresight (essential to all planning in education and social policy—a kind of 'look before you leap', 'forewarned is forearmed' behaviour).

As with the understanding of an incorporation of futures into our educational program with young children, so too the idea of globalisation. We do not need a plethora of new programs, often commercially produced, to assist us with our work with children. What is needed is a different state of mind, a new spirit and a new outlook. We have to build into everything we do with our children the perspectives of globalisation and futures. Theirs is a new world community, and children have to be participants in the planning of it.

Wortham (2001) has reported on an International Symposium on Early Childhood Education and Care held in 1999 to develop global guidelines for the education and care of young children. Some 83 early childhood professionals representing the global community met in Switzerland. An outcome of this symposium was the development of a rating scale to use in centres to categorise the strengths and weaknesses of a centre. Wortham reports that this work continues, and that the rating scale is being evaluated in a range of countries. It is hoped that this rating scale will assist a range of countries in their work on upgrading early childhood.

CHILDREN'S RIGHTS: INTO THE FUTURES

In this our final chapter, it is important to bring children's rights into focus again, this time with a futures orientation. In a Progress of Nations report (UNICEF 1994) the following was written:

> *The day will come*
> *The day will come when nations will be judged not by their military or economic*
>   *strength, nor by the splendour of their capital cities and public buildings, but:*
> *by the well being of their peoples;*
> *by their levels of health, nutrition and education;*
> *by their opportunities to earn a fair reward for their labours;*
> *by their ability to participate in the decisions that affect their lives;*
> *by the respect that is shown for their civil and political liberties;*
> *by the provision that is made for those who are vulnerable and disadvantaged;*
>   *and*
> *by the protection that is afforded to the growing minds and bodies of their*
> *children.*

Sadly, this day has not yet come. In 1995, Ebbeck wrote:

> *The belief that children have needs and rights and that childhood is special has*
> *been accepted in many developed countries although how this is translated into*
> *practice varies greatly depending on the economic, political, geographic and cul-*
> *tural context of the particular country. In many European countries, for example,*
> *childhood is celebrated and provision is made for children in all walks of life.*
> *However, in other countries children live very precariously.*   (Ebbeck 1995: 43)

In our times the world has witnessed the most horrific wars and conflicts that have inflicted death, suffering, and maiming beyond human belief. But it continues: children are often subjected not only to physical abuse but to emotional abuse as well. Well-meaning parents, who often think that they have their child's best interests and future at heart, subject very young children to an inordinate amount of stress, believing that the earlier you start formal education the better the end results!

Yet the USA, one of the world's largest democracies, was almost the last country to be a signatory (1995) to the Convention on the Rights of the Child (UNICEF 1989). Even now the U.S.A. has not yet ratified the convention so is not formally a party to it.

Anne Scheppers, a tireless campaigner for children's rights and a strong advocate, gave inspiring and challenging lectures to early childhood students at the de Lissa Institute, University of South Australia. Anne died in 2001, but the memory of her 'children's rights' approach will long be with us. Anne proposed that there is a range of views about children and their role(s) in today's world. Some people view children as the possessions of parents. Others view children as an extension of themselves. They think of their children in a kind of 'paper bag' syndrome way—to be shaken and 'carted about' in and out of shopping centres. Some see childhood as a 'stage', which children outgrow and recover from. Many see children as 'incompetent' and as needing protection, again as the property of their family. Many do not see children as citizens with rights but as entities to be exploited. Some people see that recognising the rights of children is dangerous and may break down family rights and values. They see it as a kind of see-saw model—being separate rather than inclusive members of a family with their own rights to be recognised and valued.

Anne raised the question that, if adults have a status in their own right, why is it that children do not have the same status? She believed that in many societies children are indeed marginalised and their futures insecure for a variety of reasons.

Acting on the important issues that Anne Scheppers raised we can confidently predict for now and for the future that children do have universal human rights, which must be acknowledged and met. These rights are owned by the child and are civil, political, social, cultural, economic, legal rights, which place responsibility on world governments to assist by making adequate provisions so that the child is fully prepared to live an individual life in society, and is brought up in the spirit of the ideals proclaimed in the Charter of the United Nations—in particular in the spirit of peace, dignity, tolerance, freedom, equality and solidarity (League of Nations 1924, United Nations 1959; UNICEF 1989, 1994).

This means that we have to view and treat children as persons in their own right, with needs that must be met. However, taking a children's rights perspective often does create conflict and means that early childhood professionals have a very important role to play. It also means assisting parents to see that children are not chattels or possessions. According to Kahlil Gibran (1923: 13):

> Your children are not your children
> They are the sons and daughters of Life's longing for itself.
> They come through you but not from you.
> And though they are with you yet they belong not to you.
> You may give them your love but not your thoughts
> For they have their own thoughts
> You may house their bodies but not their souls
> For their souls dwell in the house of tomorrow
> Which you cannot visit, not even in your dreams.
> You may strive to be like them, but seek not to make them like you.
> For life goes not backward nor tarries with yesterday.

What does the above mean for the early childhood professional now and for the future? In summary, it means:

- having a position on important issues;
- presenting the position verbally and in writing to government and policy makers;
- being prepared to intervene to protect the rights, dignity, health, safety and overall protection of children;
- putting children's needs first, before other interest groups;

- being a strong advocate and having input into policies so that they may be changed as needed;
- devising impact statements which show clearly the effect that a certain policy or action will have on the lives of children;
- making sure that policies are articulated and fit positively together;
- being accountable and responsible in relation to advocacy;
- being a watchdog for the profession;
- being constantly alert to any development in the policy area that has the potential to adversely affect the quality of life for children;
- at all times implementing an early childhood code of ethical practice; and
- being futures-oriented in considering the potential impact on children of a certain global issue or trend, and being proactive in relation to the rights of the child when and as needed.

Harvey, Dolgopol and Castel-McGregor (1993:3) proposed that people working in the area of or with an interest in children's rights should learn how to use the Convention on the Rights of the Child (1989) as a lobbying tool and should consider the implications of this in their own specific work. This is sound practical advice and should be considered in relation to the issues on implementing policies raised in Chapter 5. Likewise, Nicol (1992: 15) had some relevant points to make:

> In the final analysis decisions are best made based on internationally agreed standards. An example of such an initiative is when staff, parents, school managers and community members can be involved in drawing up their own Children's Charter based on these. In the UK for instance the Children Act (1989) enshrines many of the recommendations of the UN Convention on the Rights of the Child (1989). In particular it echoes the ideal that all decisions should be made in the child's best interests, not the school's or the parent's. It also gives the child a voice in major decisions such as choosing which school she wants to attend.

This statement by Nicol is a timely reminder that children's voices need to be heard and that they can sometimes be overlooked even when it comes to decisions affecting their life now and for the future. There is an old proverb that says 'It's better to build children than repair adults'. Government in their futures charters should give cognisance to this.

To return to the theme of globalisation, globalisation requires us, as administrators, managers and leaders in early childhood, to respect the values and cultures of the people, the children and the families with whom we work. Curricula also have to be acceptable and unbiased. Our goal is, as said before, to help all young children with whom we work to become leaders within their own local culture, even though they are part of a much larger society and culture.

Grey (1999: 1) reminds us that a vision is a realistic, credible, attractive future which has the power to energise all involved to commit themselves to the pursuit of excellence. This statement of Grey's challenges us to articulate a vision for the future, one which assists early childhood centres and schools in achieving excellence. This vision needs to take cognisance of globalisation and the future world trends in education that are likely to affect early childhood education.

Likewise, Stonehouse (1998a, b) remains optimistic about the future for children, for children's services and for the professions. However, she emphasises the need to be political and to be advocates—wise words for the future!

CHAPTER SUMMARY

This chapter has attempted to present the complex concepts of globalisation and futures, and what these might mean to teachers and early childhood leaders.

- Some managers seek simple and easy solutions to what are often difficult problems.
- Changing the attitude and mindset of anyone is not an easy task. What we have been discussing in this chapter is just that—the changing of the attitudes and mindsets of the children, their teachers and educational managers as these relate to issues of globalisation and futures. In one sense the solution could be seen as simple—that is, if only the teachers were themselves to have a futures and global perspective.
- The responsibility for the curriculum in a classroom rests, in the main, with the classroom teacher. Even where the curriculum is a centralised one, the way it is implemented (taught), the emphases and nuances made by the teacher and so on, can overcome to a large degree any conformity that might be inherent in such a curriculum.
- So a large part of the responsibility for changing the way children behave towards their learning has to rest with the teacher and the educational manager, be this the school/centre principal or curriculum specialist.
- The same can be said about leadership: the responsibility for taking staff further is a part of the leader's responsibilities and accountabilities.
- The leader must be a visionary and have the ability to help others share in visions of the future and to enthuse all to be part of this futures-oriented thinking.
- The chapter has presented the visions of some forward-thinking, well-known early childhood educators. It is worth giving serious consideration to their views, as these are based on experience, knowledge and a commitment to the field of early childhood.

Discussion and reflection

1. Note down your understanding of the terms 'globalisation' and 'futures'.

    (a) What influences do you see acting on the futures of early childhood education?
    (b) What changes would you forecast for the next five years? How positive or negative are these changes likely to be?
    (c) What are some strategies you could use as an early childhood leader in order to be proactive in coping with the likely effects of globalisation?
    (d) What are some of the problems that early childhood personnel may face in implementing a visionary future for their own particular early childhood centre?
    (e) Note down your own Nostradamus predictions, as Bettye Caldwell has done in this chapter.
    (f) How do your predictions differ from those presented in extracts in this chapter?

Bibliography

Adam, J. 1991, *Employer sponsored child care: An issues paper*, Community Child Care, Melbourne.

Almy, M. 1975, *The early childhood educator at work*, McGraw-Hill, New York.

Al-Otaibi, M. 1997, 'Accreditation of early CE in the USA: a model for Saudi Arabia?', *Child Study Journal* vol. 27, no. 3, pp. 191–219.

Andersson, B.E. 1992, 'Effects of day care on cognitive and socio-emotional competence of thirteen year old Swedish schoolchildren', *Child Development*, no. 63, pp. 20–36.

Ashton, J. & Cairney, T. 2001, 'Understanding the discourses of partnership: an examination of one school's attempt at parent involvement', *Australian Journal of Language and Literacy*, vol. 24, no. 2, pp. 145–55.

Atkinson, A.M. 1991, 'Fathers' participation in day care', *Early Child Development and Care*, vol. 66, pp. 115–26.

Australian Early Childhood Association (AECA) 1997, *National Newsletter*, no. 2, pp. 4–5.

Barclay, K. & Benelli, C. 1996, 'Program evaluation through the eyes of a child', *Childhood Education*, no. 72, pp. 91–6.

Barnard, C.I. 1938, *Functions of the Executive*, Harvard University Press, Cambridge, MA.

Barth, J.M. & Parker, R.D. 1993, 'Parent-child relationship influences in children's transition to school', *Merrill-Palmer Quarterly*, vol. 39, no. 2, pp. 173–95.

Beare, H. & Slaughter, R. 1994, *Education for the twenty-first century*, Routledge, London.

Bell, J. & Harrison, B.T. 1998, *Leading people: Learning from people. Lessons from education professionals*, OUP, Philadelphia, PA.

Bellamy, C. 2002, *The state of the world's children 2002: Leadership*, United Nations Children's Fund, Paris
(http://www.unicef.org/sowc02/pdf/sowc2002-final-eng-allmod.txt).

Bennis, W.G., Benne, K.D. & Chin, R. 1985, *The planning of change*, 4th edn, Holt, Rinehart & Winston, New York.

Berk, L. 2000, *Child Development*, Allyn & Bacon, Boston.

Bhavangari, N.P. & Gonzalez-Mena, J. 1997, 'The cultural context of infant caregiving'. *Childhood Education*, vol. 75, pp. 2–8.

Biggs, S. 1989, *Corporate child care: The bottom-line conference papers*, Child Care at Work, Sydney.

Blank, H.K. 1997, 'Advocacy leadership', in *Leadership in early care and education*, S.L. Kagan & B. Bowman (eds), NAEYC, Washington, DC, pp. 39–45.

Bolton, R. 1986, *People skills: How to assert yourself, listen to others, and resolve conflicts*, Prentice-Hall, Sydney.

Boutte, G.S., Keepler, D.L., Tyler, V.S. & Terry, B.Z. 1992, 'Effective techniques for involving "difficult" parents', *Young Children*, vol. 47, no. 3, pp. 19–22.

Bredekamp, S. 1999, 'When new solutions create new problems: Lessons learned from NAEYC accreditation', *Young Children*, vol. 54, no. 1, pp. 58–63.

Brennan, D. 1998a, *The politics of Australian child care: Philanthropy to feminism and beyond*, revised edn, Cambridge University Press, Melbourne.

Brennan, D. 1998b, 'Counterpoint: Child care reform and labour market participation by women', *Australian Journal of Early Childhood*, vol. 23, no. 3, pp. 5–7.

Bridgman, P. & Davis, G. 1998, *Australian policy handbook*, Allen & Unwin, Sydney.

Broinowski, I. 1994, *Managing of child care centres*, TAFE Publications, Melbourne.

Bronfenbrenner, U. 1979, *The ecology of human development: Experiments by nature and design*, Harvard University Press, Cambridge.

Bronfenbrenner, U. & Weiss, H.B. 1983, 'Beyond policies without people: an ecological perspective on child and family policy', in *Children, families and government: Perspectives on American social policy*, E.F. Zigler, S.L. Kagan & E. Klugman (eds), Cambridge University Press, London.

Brooker, L. 2001, 'Interviewing children', in *Doing early childhood research: International perspectives on theory and practice*, G. MacNaughton, S. Rolfe & I. Siraj-Blatchford (eds), Allen & Unwin, Sydney, pp. 162–77.

Buell, M.J. & Cassidy, D.J. 2001, 'The complexity and dynamic nature of quality in early care and educational programs: A case for chaos theory', *Journal of Research in Childhood Education*, vol. 15, no. 2, pp. 209–19.

Burchinal, M.R., Roberts, J.E., Riggins, R. Jr., Zeisel, S.A., Neebe, E. & Bryant, D. 2000, 'Relating quality of centre based child care to early cognitive and language development longitudinally', *Child Development*, vol. 71, no. 2, pp. 339–57.

Burns, R. 1993, *Managing people in changing times*, Allen & Unwin, Sydney.

Burton, J. & Dukes, F. (eds) 1990, *Conflict: readings in management and resolution*, St Martin's Press, New York.

Butterworth, D. & Candy, J. 1998, 'Quality early childhood practice for young Aboriginal children', *Australian Journal of Early Childhood*, vol. 23, no. 2, pp. 20–5.

Cairney, T. 1997, 'Parents and literacy learning: New perspectives', *Every Child*, vol. 3, no. 2, pp. 4–5.

Caldwell, B.M. 1983, 'How can we educate the American public about the child care profession?', *Young Children*, March, pp. 11–17.

Carter, M. 2000, 'Considering our curriculum in working with families: Ideas for training staff', *Child Care Information Exchange*, no. 134, pp. 90–3.

Carter, M. & Curtis, D. 1998, *The visionary director: A handbook for dreaming, organising and improvising in your centre*, Redleaf Press, St Paul, MN.

Caughy, M.O., DiPietro, J.A. & Strobino, D.M. 1994, 'Day care participation as a protective factor in the cognitive development of low-income children', *Child Development*, no. 65, pp. 457–71.

Chapman, E. & O'Neil, S.L. 2000, *Leadership: Essential steps every manager needs to know*, Prentice Hall, Upper Saddle River, NJ.

Chin, R., Bennis, W.G. & Benne, K.D. 1961, *The planning of change*, Holt, Rinehart & Winston, New York.

Chomsky, N. 1994, *Keeping the rabble in line: Interviews with David Barsamian*, AK Press, Edinburgh.

Chomsky, N. 1996, *Power and prospects: Reflections on human nature and the social order*, Allen & Unwin, Sydney.

Clark-Stewart, K.A. 1987, 'Predicting child development from childcare forms and features: The Chicago study', in *Quality in child care: What does the research tell us?*, D. Phillips (ed.), NAEYC, Washington, DC.

Clyde, M., Parmenter, G., Rodd, J., Rolfe, S., Tinworth, S. & Waniganayake, M. 1994, 'Child care from the perspective of parents, caregivers and children: Australian research', in *Advances in Early Education and Day Care*, S. Reifel (ed.), JAI Press, Greenwich, pp. 189–234.

Colebatch, H.K. 1998, *Policy*, Open University Press, Buckingham.

Cost Quality and Child Outcomes Study team 1995, *Cost, quality and child outcomes in child care centres. A Public Report, (2nd edn)*, Denver Department of Economics, University of Colorado, Denver.

Cox, E. 1995, *A truly civil society*, Boyer Lectures. Australian Broadcasting Corporation, Sydney.

Cox, E. 1996, *Leading women: Tactics for making the difference*, Random House, Sydney.

Crawley, J. 1992, *Constructive conflict management: Managing to make a difference*, Nicholas Brealey Publishing, London.

Crompton, D.A. 1997, 'Community leadership', in *Leadership in early care and education*, S.L. Kagan & B. Bowman (eds), NAEYC, Washington, DC, pp. 49–55.

Cryer, D. 1999, 'Defining and assessing early childhood program quality', *The Annals of the American Academy of Political and Social Science*, no. 563, pp. 39–55.

Cryer, D. & Phillipsen, L. 1997, 'Quality details: A close look at child care programs and strengths and weaknesses', *Young Children*, vol. 52, no. 5, pp. 51–61.

Curriculum Corporation 1993, *Curriculum Statements and Profiles*, Melbourne, Victoria.

de Lemos, M. & Mellor, E. 1994, 'A longitudinal study of developmental maturity, school entry age and school progress', *Journal of Australian Research in Early Childhood Education*, vol. 1, pp. 42–50.

Deater-Deckard, K., Pinkerton, R. & Scarr, S. 1996, 'Child care quality and children's behavioural adjustment: a four year longitudinal study', *Journal of Child Psychology & Psychiatry*, vol. 37, no. 8, pp. 937–48.

Decker, C. & Decker, J. 1984, *Planning and administering early childhood programs*, 3rd edn, Merrill, Columbus, OH.

Decker, C. & Decker, J. 1988, *Planning and administering early childhood programs*, 4th edn, Merrill/Prentice Hall, Upper Saddle River, NJ.

Department of Education and Children's Services (DECS) 1996, *Foundation areas of learning*, DECS, Adelaide.

Department of Education and Children's Services 1997, *Foundations for the future: A declaration for South Australian public education and children's services*, DECS, Adelaide.

Department of Education Training and Employment (DETE) 1998, *South Australian Curriculum, Standards and Accountability Framework, Implementation Plan*, DETE, Adelaide.

Department of Education Training and Employment 2001, *South Australian Curriculum, Standards and Accountability Framework* [On-line, accessed 1 June 2002] (URL: http:// www.sacsa.sa.edu.au).

Dewey, J. 1933, *How we think. A restatement of the relation of reflective thinking to the educative process*, DC Heath, Chicago, Illinois.

Dockett, S. & Perry, B. (eds) 2001, *Beginning school together: Sharing strengths*, AECA, Canberra.

Doherty-Derkowski, G. 1995, *Quality matters: Excellence in early childhood programs*, Addison-Wesley, Don Mills, Ontario.

Duff, R.E., Brown, M.H. & Van Scoy, I.J. 1995, 'Reflection and self evaluation: Key to professional development', *Young Children*, vol. 50, no. 4, pp. 81–8.

Duggan, E. 2002, 'Pace of change worsens teaching stress problems', *The Australian*, 8–9 June, p. 11.

Dunphy, D. 1986, *Organisational change by choice*, Prentice Hall, Sydney.

Ebbeck, F.N. 2001, *ERIC Clearing House: Quality is culture-bound* [On-line, accessed 14 Mar. 2002] (URL: http://ericeece.org).

Ebbeck, M. 1991, *Early childhood education*, Longman Cheshire, Melbourne.

Ebbeck, M. 1995, 'The rights of the child—theory into practice', *Early Child Development and Care*, vol. 112, pp. 43–52.

Ebbeck, M. 1997, 'Parents as arbiters of quality in child care', *Gowrie News*, Spring, pp. 10–11.

Ebbeck, M. & Clyde, M. 1988, 'Early childhood teaching: The disintegrated profession?', *Early Childhood Development and Care*, vol. 34, pp. 279–85.

Ebbeck, M. & Ebbeck, F. 1994, 'Accountability and the early childhood profession', *Australian Journal of Early Childhood*, vol. 19, no. 1, pp. 16–20.

Ebbeck, M. & Glover, A. 1998, 'Immigrant families' expectations of early childhood', *Australian Journal of Early Childhood*, vol. 23, no. 3, pp. 9–13.

Eisenberg, E. & Rafanello, D. 1998, 'Accreditation facilitation: a study of one project's success', *Young Children*, vol. 53, no. 5, pp. 44–8.

Elliott, A. 2000a, 'Shaping early childhood futures: Visions for children, families and communities', *Every Child*, vol. 6, no. 3, Spring, p. 3.

Elliott, A. 2000b, 'Visions of children and childhood', *Every Child*, vol. 6, no. 3, pp. 6–7.

Emblen, V. 1998, 'Providers and families: Do they have the same views of early childhood programmes? Some questions realised by working on early childhood education in the Lao Peoples Democratic Republic', *International Journal of Early Childhood*, vol. 30, pp. 31–7.

Epstein, J.L. 1995, 'School/family/community partnerships: Caring for the children we share', *Phi Delta Kappa*, vol. 76, no. 9, pp. 701–12.

Epstein, J.L. & Sanders, M.G. 1998, 'What we learn from international studies of school-family-community partnerships', *Childhood Education*, vol. 74, no. 6, pp. 392–4.

Farmer, S. 1995, *Policy development in early childhood services*, Community Child Care Cooperative, Sydney.

Fenna, A. 1998, *Introduction to Australian public policy*, Longman, Melbourne.

Fish, S. 1991, 'But can you prove it? Quality assurance and the reflective practitioner', *Assessment and Evaluation in Higher Education*, vol. 16, no. 1, pp. 22–36.

Fleer, M. 1996, 'Early childhood science education: Acknowledging and valuing differing cultural understandings', *Australian Journal of Early Childhood*, vol. 21, no. 3, pp. 11–15.

Fleet, A. & Clyde, M. 1993, *What's in a day? Working in early childhood*, Social Science Press, Wentworth Falls, NSW.

Foster, J.E. & Loven, R.G. 1992, 'The need and directions for parent involvement in the 1990s. Undergraduate perspectives and expectation', *Action for Teacher Education*, vol. 14, pp. 13–18.

Fullan, M.G. 1982, *The meaning of educational change*, Teachers College Press, New York.

Fullan, M.G. 1991, *The new meaning of educational change*, 2nd edn, Cassell, London.

Fullan, M. & Hargreaves, A. (eds) 1992, *Teacher development and educational change*, Falmer Press, London, NY.

Gallinsky, E. 1988, 'Parents and teacher-caregivers: Sources of tension, sources of support', *Young Children*, vol. 43, no. 3, pp. 4–12.

Gallinsky, E. 1990, 'Why are some parent/teacher partnerships clouded with difficulties?', *Young Children*, vol. 45, no. 5, pp. 2–3, 38–9.

Gellens, S. 1998, 'Involving parents and teachers in the evaluation process', *Child Care Information Exchange*, vol. 75, no. 123, pp. 92–7.

Gestwicki, C. 1992, *Home, school and community relations*, Delmar Publishers, Albany, NY.

Gibran, K. 1923, *The Prophet*, Heinemann, London.

Goelman, H. & Guo, H. 1998, 'What we know and what we don't know about burnout among early childhood care providers', *Child & Youth Care Forum*, vol. 27, no. 3, June, pp. 175–99.

Goffin, S.G. & Lombardi, J. 1988, *Speaking out: Early childhood advocacy*, NAEYC, Washington, DC.

Goh, C.T. 1999, *Straits Times*, 20 November.

Gonzalez-Mena, J. 1992, 'Taking a culturally sensitive approach in infant-toddler programs', *Young Children*, vol. 47, no. 2, pp. 4–9.

Gormley, W. 1997, *Everybody's children*, The Brookings Institute, Washington, DC.

Gormley, W. 1999, 'Regulating child care quality', *Annals of the American Academy of Political and Social Science*, no. 563, pp. 116–29.

Goward, P. 2002, *Valuing parenthood: Options for paid maternity leave, an interim paper*, Sex discrimination Unit, Human Rights and Equal Opportunity Commission, Sydney.

Grey, A.E. 1999, 'A vision of quality in early childhood education', *Australian Journal of Early Childhood*, vol. 24, no. 3, September, pp. 1–4.

Grieshaber, S. 2000, 'Regulating the early childhood field', *Australian Journal of Early Childhood*, vol. 25, no. 2, pp. 1–6.

Gullo, D.F. & Burton, C.B. 1993, 'The effects of social class, class size and prekinder-garten experience on early school adjustment', *Early Child Development and Care*, vol. 88, pp. 43–51.

Hagekull, B. & Bohlin, G. 1995, 'Day care quality, family and child characteristics and socio-emotional development', *Early Childhood Research Quarterly*, no. 10, pp. 505–26.

Handy, C. 1932, *The Age of Unreason*, Hutchinson Business, London.

Harms, T. & Clifford, R. 1980, *The Early Childhood Environment Rating Scale (ECERS)*, Teachers College Press, New York.

Harm, T., Clifford, R. & Cryer, D. 1998, Early Childhood Environment Rating Scale-Revised Edition (ECERS-R), Teachers College Press, New York.

Harrison, L. & Ungerer, J.A. 1997, 'Child care predictors of infant-mother attachment security at age 12 months', *Early Child Development and Care*, vol. 137, pp. 31–46.

Harvey, J., Dolgopol, U. & Castell-Mcgregor (eds) 1993, *Implementing the UN Convention on the Rights of the Child in Australia*, Children's Interest Bureau, Adelaide.

Hasenfeld, Y. 1983, *Human service organisations*, Prentice Hall, Englewood Cliffs, NJ.

Hayden, J. 1996, *Management of early childhood services: An Australian perspective*, Social Science Press, Sydney.

Hayden, J. 1994, 'The public image of child care', *Every Child*, Spring, 1: 14–16.

Hayden, J. 1999, *Delegation*, Australian Early Childhood Association, Canberra.

Hayden, J. (ed.) 2000, *Landscapes in early childhood education: Cross-national perspectives on empowerment—a guide for the new millennium*, Peter Lang, New York.

Hayes, A. & Press, F. 2000, *OECD thematic review of early childhood education and care policy*, Commonwealth of Australia, Canberra.

Hays, T., Gerber, R. & Minichiello, V. 1999, 'Mentorship: A review of the concept', *Unicorn*, vol. 25, no. 2, pp. 84–95.

Herr, J., Johnson, D.R. & Zimmerman, K. 1993, 'Benefits of accreditation: A study of directors' perceptions', *Young Children*, vol. 48, no. 4, pp. 32–5.

Hildebrand, V. & Hearron, P. 1997, 'Monitoring and controlling for quality', in *Management of child development centres*, Merrill, Columbus, OH, pp. 190–211.

Hill, M. 1989, 'The role of social networks in the care of young children', *Children and Society*, vol. 3, no. 3, pp. 195–211.

Hodge, B.J. & Johnson, H.J. 1988, 'Management and organizational behavior', in B.J. Hodge & W.P. Anthony 1988, *Organization theory*, 3rd edn, Allyn & Bacon, Boston, MA.

Hornibrook, M.& Wallace, M. (n.d.), Executive Summary, *Report on the Independent Evaluation of the Development of the South Australian Curriculum, Standards and Accountability Framework*, Curriculum Corporation, Adelaide.

Howes, C. 1983, 'Caregiver behaviour in centres and in family day care', *Journal of Applied Developmental Psychology*, no. 4, pp. 99–107.

Howes, C. & Rubenstein, J. 1985, 'Determinants of toddlers' experiences in day care: Age of entry and quality of setting', *Child Care Quarterly*, vol. 14, no. 2, pp. 140–51.

Hughes, P. & MacNaughton, G. 1999, 'Who's the expert: Reconceptualising parent-staff relation in early education', *Australian Journal of Early Childhood*, vol. 24, no. 4, pp. 27–32.

Hughes, P. & MacNaughton, G. 2000, 'Consensus, dissensus or community: The politics of parent involvement in early childhood education', *Contemporary Issues in Early Childhood*, vol. 1, no. 3, pp. 241–58.

Hujala, E. & Puroila, A. (eds) 1998, *Towards understanding leadership in early childhood context: Cross-cultural perspectives*, Oulu University Press, Oulu, Finland.

Hujala-Huutunen, E. 1996, 'Day care in the USA, Russia and Finland: Views from parents, teachers and directors', *European Early Childhood Education Research Journal*, vol. 4, no. 1, pp. 33–47.

Hydon, C. 2002, 'RRRC: real rights for refugee children', *Australian Early Childhood Association, Victoria Branch, Newsletter*, vol. 6, no. 1, p. 7.

Jacobs, N.L. 1992, 'Unhappy endings', *Young Children*, vol. 47, no. 3, pp. 23–7.

Jalongo, M.R. & Isenberg, J.P. 2000, *Exploring your role: A practitioner's introduction to early childhood education*, Merrill/Prentice Hall, Columbus, OH.

Jalongo, M.R. & Mutuku, M.M. 1999, 'Monitoring quality without sacrificing substance', in *Resisting the pendulum swing: Informed perspectives on education controversies*, M.R. Jalongo (ed.), ACEI, Olney, MD, pp. 125–33.

Jayatilaka, J. 2001, 'Family literacy: Schools and families of young children working together', *Australian Journal of Early Childhood*, vol. 26, no. 2, pp. 20–4.

Jensen, M.A. & Hannibal, M.A.Z. 2000, *Issues, advocacy, and leadership in early education*, 2nd edn, Allyn & Bacon, London.

Jensen, R.A. & Kiley, R.J. 2000, *Teaching, leading, and learning: Becoming caring professionals*, Houghton Mifflin, New York.

Johnson, L.J., LaMontagne, M.J., Elgas, P.M. & Bauer, A.M. 1998, *Early childhood education: Blending theory, blending practice*, Paul H. Brookes Publishing, Baltimore, MD.

Jones, A. & May, J. 1997, *Working in human service organisations: A critical introduction*, Longman, Melbourne.

Jorde-Bloom, P. 1982, *Avoiding burnout: Strategies for managing time, space and people in early childhood education*, Acropolis House, Washington, DC.

Jorde-Bloom, P. 1995, 'Shared decision-making: The centre piece of participatory management', *Young Children*, vol. 50, no. 4, pp. 55–60.

Jorde-Bloom, P. 1997, 'Commentary', in *Leadership in Early Care and Education*, S. Kagan & T. Bowman (eds), NAEYC, Washington, DC, pp. 34–7.

Jorde-Bloom, P., Sheerer, M. & Britz, J. 1991a, Blue print for action. Achieving centre-based change through staff development. New Horizons, Mt Rainier, MD.

Jorde-Bloom, P., Sheerer, M. & Britz, J. 1991b, 'Leadership style assessment tool', *Child Care Information Exchange*, Oct., no. 87, pp. 12–15.

Kagan, S.L. 1994, 'Leadership: Rethinking it—making it happen', *Young Children*, vol. 49, no. 5, pp. 50–4.

Kagan, S. & Bowman, T. (eds) 1997, *Leadership in Early Care and Education*, NAEYC, Washington, DC.

Kagan, S.L. & Rivera, A.M. 1991, 'Collaboration in early care and education: What can and should we expect?', *Young Children*, vol. 47, no. 1, pp. 51–6.

Kamerman, S.B. & Kahn, A.J. 1987, *The responsive workplace: Employers and a changing workplace*, Columbus University Press, New York.

Kaplan, M.G. & Conn, J.S. 1984, 'The effects of caregiver training on classroom setting and caregiver performance in eight community day care centres', *Child Study Journal*, vol. 14, no. 2, pp. 79–93.

Karrby, G. 1999, 'Conceptions of quality in early childhood education: An analysis of rationales for the rating of quality with the ECERs', paper presented to European Early Childhood Education Research Association's 9th Conference, Helsinki, 1–4 Sept.

Kasting, A. 1994, 'Respect, responsibility and reciprocity: The 3 Rs of parent involvement', *Childhood Education*, vol. 70, no. 3, pp. 146–50.

Katz, L. 1995, *Talks with teachers of young children: A collection*, Ablex Publishing, New Jersey.

Katz, L. & Bauch, J. 1999, 'The Peabody Family involvement initiative. Preparing preservice teachers for family/school collaboration activities', *School Community Journal*, vol. 9, no. 1, pp. 49–69.

Keary, A. 2000, 'Changing images of mother/mothering', *Australian Journal of Early Childhood*, vol. 25, no. 2, pp. 13–17.

Kelly, J. 1992, 'Voluntary accreditation: The New South Wales experience', *Australian Journal of Early Childhood*, vol. 17, no. 1, pp. 10–16.

Kimbrough, R.B. & Nunnery, M.Y. 1998, *Educational administration: An introduction*, 3rd edn, Macmillan, New York.

Kincheloe, J.L. 1993, *Toward a critical politics of teacher thinking. Mapping the postmodern*, Bergin and Garvey, Westport, Connecticut.

Kirner, J. & Rayner, M. 1999, *The women's power handbook: Get it, keep it, use it*, Viking/Penguin, Melbourne.

Kontos, S. & Stremmel, A.J. 1988, 'Caregiver's perceptions of working conditions in a child care environment', *Early Childhood Research Quarterly*, no. 3, pp. 77–90.

Kotter, J.P. 1990, 'What leaders really do', *Harvard Business Review*, May–June, pp. 103–11.

Langford, J. & Weissbourd, B. 1997, 'New directions for parent leadership in a family support context', in *Leadership in early care and education*, S.L. Kagan & B.T. Bowman (eds), NAEYC, Washington, DC, pp. 147–53.

Langsted, O. 1994, 'Looking at quality from the child's perspective', in *Valuing quality in early childhood services*, P. Moss & A. Pence (eds), Paul Chapman Publishing, London, pp. 28–42.

League of Nations 1924, *The Declaration of the Rights of the Child*, League of Nations, Geneva.

Lewin, K. 1935, *A dynamic theory of personality*, McGraw-Hill, London, NY.

Loane, S. 1997, *Who cares? Guilt, hope and the child care debate*, Mandarin, Sydney.

Lyons, M. 1996, 'Who cares? Child care, trade unions and staff turnover', *Journal of Industrial Relations*, vol. 38, pp. 629–47.

Lyons, M. 1997, 'Work rewards, job satisfaction and accreditation in long day care', *Australian Journal of Early Childhood*, vol. 22, no. 3, pp. 40–4.

Macpherson, A. 1993, 'Parent-professional partnership: A review and discussion of issues', *Early Child Development and Care*, no. 86, pp. 61–77.

Magill, E. 1993, 'Formulating policies for a new centre', *Rattler*, no. 25, Autumn, p. 24.

Margetts, K. 2002, *Child care arrangements, personal, family and school influences on children's adjustment to the first year of schooling* [On-line, accessed June 2002]. (URL: http://www.edfac.unimelb.edu.au/child_care).

Marriott, P. 2001, *Child care: Beyond 2001*, a report for the Minister for Family and Community Services and the Commonwealth Child Care Advisory Council, Canberra.

Meredith, H., Perry, B., Borg, T. & Dockett, S. 1999, 'Changes in parents' perceptions of their children's transition to school: First child and later children', *Journal of Australian Research in Early Childhood Education*, vol. 6, no. 2, pp. 228–30.

Ministry of Education Singapore 1999a, *Speech by RADM (NS) Teo Chee Hean, Minister for Education and Second Minister for Defence at SINDA's 8th Academic Excellence Awards Ceremony on 30 October 1999* [On-line, accessed 3 Nov. 2001] (URL: http://www.moe.edu.sg/speeches/1999/sp301099.htm).

Ministry of Education Singapore 1999b, *Committee to Study Compulsory Education* [On-line, accessed 4 Nov. 2001] (URL: http://www.moe.edu.sg/press/1999/pr991221a.htm).

Ministry of Education Singapore 2000a, *Aline Wong Committee Recommends Compulsory Primary Education* [On-line, accessed 3 Nov. 2001] (URL: http://www.moe.edu.sg/press/2000/pr15082000.htm).

Ministry of Education Singapore 2000b, *Opening Speech by RADM (NS) Teo Chee Hean, Minister for Education and Second Minister for Defence at the Second Reading of the Compulsory Education Bill on 9 October 2000* [On-line, accessed 3 Nov. 2001] (URL: http://www.moe.edu.sg/speeches/2000/sp09102000.htm).

Ministry of Education Singapore 2000c, *Closing Speech by RADM (NS) Teo Chee Hean, Minister for Education and Second Minister for Defence at the Second Reading of the Compulsory education Bill on 9 October 2000* [On-line, accessed 3 Nov. 2001] (URL: http://www.moe.edu.sg/speeches/2000/sp09102000a.htm).

Ministry of Education Singapore 2000d, *Speech by RADM (NS) Teo Chee Hean, Minister for Education and Second Minister for Defence at the Edusave Merit Bursary/Edusave Scholarship/CDC-CCC on 31 December 2000* [On-line, accessed 4 Nov. 2001] (URL: http://www.moe.edu.sg/speeches/2000/sp31122000.htm).

Ministry of Education Singapore 2000e, *Compulsory Education Report* [On-line, accessed 3 Nov. 2001] (URL: http://www.moe.edu.sg/press/2000/ce_report.pdf).

Mitchell, J. 1990, *Revisioning educational leadership: A phenomenological approach*, Bergin & Garvey, New York.

Mohan, T., McGregor, H. & Strano, Z. 1992, *Communicating theory and practice*, 3rd edn, Harcourt Brace Jovanovich, Sydney.

Morgan, G. 1997, 'Historical views of leadership', in *Leadership in early care and education*, S. Kagan & T. Bowman (eds), NAEYC, Washington, DC, pp. 9–14.

Moss, P. & Pence, A. (eds) 1994, *Valuing quality in early childhood services*, Paul Chapman, London.

Murray, S. 1996, 'Evaluating the evaluation of child care accreditation', *Australian Journal of Early Childhood*, vol. 21, no. 2, pp. 12–16.

National Association for the Education of Young Children (NAEYC) 1993, *A conceptual framework for early childhood professional development*, NAEYC, Washington, DC.

National Association for the Education of Young Children 1996, 'Be a children's champion', *Young Children*, January, pp. 58–60.

National Association for the Education of Young Children 1999, *A conceptual framework for early childhood professional development*, NAEYC, Washington, DC.

National Association of Community Based Children's Services (NACBCS) 2001, *Children First Campaign: Your personal lobby kit*, NACBCS Secretariat, Community Child Care Victoria, Melbourne.

National Childcare Accreditation Council (NCAC) 1993, *Putting children first: Quality Improvement and Accreditation System Handbook*, 1st edn, NCAC, Sydney.

National Childcare Accreditation Council 2001a, *Choosing quality child care*, NCAC, Sydney.

National Childcare Accreditation Council 2001b, *Quality Improvement and Accreditation System Handbook*, 2nd edn, NCAC, Sydney (URL: http://www.ncac.gov.au).

Neugebauer, R. & Neugebauer, B. (eds) 1998, *The art of leadership: Managing early childhood organizations*, vol. 2, Child Care Information Exchange, Perth.

Ng, H.K., Gan, S.-L. & Menon, J. 2001, 'Newspaper reporting and children's television programming in Singapore', in *Children in the news: Reporting of children's issues in television and the press in Asia*, Asian Media Information and Communication Center (AMIC)/School of Communication Studies, Nanyang Technological University, Singapore, pp. 302–52.

Nicol, E. 1992, 'The European dimension, internalisation, education for citizenship and human rights in the early years', *Early Years*, vol. 12, no. 2, pp. 13–17.

Nilsen, B. 1997, *Week by week: Plans for observing and recording young children*, Delmar Publishers, Albany, NY.

Nivala, V. 1998, 'Theoretical perspectives on educational leadership', in *Towards understanding leadership in early childhood context: Cross-cultural perspectives*, E. Hujala & A. Puriola (eds), Oulu University Press, Oulu, Finland, pp. 49–62.

Noone, M. 1996, *Mediation*, Cavendish Publishing, London.

Nupponen, H. 2000, 'Leadership and management into the 21st century, *Every Child*, vol. 6, no. 3, pp. 8–9.

Oberhuemer, P. 2000, 'Conceptualising the professional role in early childhood centres: Emerging profiles in four European countries', *Early Childhood Research and Practice* [Electronic], vol. 2, no. 2, pp. 1–3, Available [2002, Aug. 15] (http://ecrp.uiuc.edu/v2n2/oberhuemer).

Ochiltree, G. 1994, *Effects of child care on young children. Forty years of research*, *Early Childhood Study Paper no. 5*, Australian Institute of Family Studies, Melbourne.

Olmsted, P.P. 1994, 'Families speak', in *The IEA Preprimary Project Phare 1: Early childhood care and education and care in 11 countries. Research Report no. 143*, D.P. Weikart (ed.), D. High/Scope Press, Ypsilanti, MI.

Organization for Economic Cooperation and Development (OECD) 2001, *Starting Strong: Early childhood education and care. Education and skills*, OECD Publications, Paris (http://oecdpublications.gfi-nb.com/cgi-bin/oecdbookshop.storefront).

Page, J., Niehuys, T., Kapsalakis, A. & Morda, R. 2001, 'Parents' perceptions of kindergarten programs in Victoria', *Australian Journal of Early Childhood*, vol. 26, no. 3, pp. 43–50.

Palmer, G. 2000, 'Resilience in child refugees. An historical study', *Australian Journal of Early Childhood*, vol. 25, no. 3, pp. 39–45.

Patten, C. 1998, *East and West*, Macmillan, London.

Peltonen, J. & Halonen, T. 1998, 'Two conceptions of action research: A continuation of traditional social research and a new, critical social science', in *Towards understanding leadership in early childhood context: Cross-cultural perspectives*, E. Hujala & A. Puroila (eds), Oulu University Press, Oulu, pp. 79–92.

Pence, A. & Moss, P. (eds) 1994, *Valuing quality in early childhood services*, Paul Chapman, London.

Petrie, A. 1992, 'Chasing ideologies: The past is still before us', in *Changing faces: The early childhood profession in Australia*, B. Lambert (ed.), Australian Early Childhood Association, Canberra, pp. 12–30.

Phillips, D. (ed.) 1987, *Quality in child care: What does the research tell us?*, NAEYC, Washington, DC.

Phillips, D., Howes, C. & Whitebook, M. 1991, 'Child care as an adult work environment', *Journal of Social Issues*, vol. 47, no. 2, pp. 49–70.

Powell, D. 1989, *Families and early childhood programs. Resource monograph no. 3*, NAEYC, Washington, DC.

Press, F. 1999, 'The demise of community owned long day care centres and the rise of the mythical consumer', *Australian Journal of Early Childhood*, vol. 24, no. 1, pp. 20–5.

Press, F. & Hayes, A. 2000, *OECD thematic review of early childhood education and care: Australian background report*, Commonwealth of Australia, Canberra.

Public Policy Report 1996, *Young Children*, vol. 51, no. 2, pp. 58–60.

Puckett, M., Marshall, C.S. & Davis, R. 1999, 'Examining the emergence of brain development research: The promises and the perils', *Childhood Education*, Fall, pp. 8–12.

Pugh, G. (ed.) 1996, *Contemporary issues in the early years*, Paul Chapman, London.

Pungello, E., Campbell, F.A. & Miller-Johnson, S. 2000, 'Benefits of high quality child-care for low-income mothers: The Abecedarian Study', paper presented to Head Start National Research Conference, Washington, DC, 28 Jun.–1 Jul.

Putnam, R.D. 1995, 'Bowling alone: America's declining social capital', *Journal of Democracy*, January, pp. 65–78.

Raban, B. 2000, *Just the beginning . . .* A report prepared as the Inaugural DETYA Research Fellow 1999–2000, Research and Evaluation Branch, Department of Education, Training and Youth Affairs, Canberra.

Raban, B.B. 2001, 'Reading in early childhood and developing literacy', *Australian Journal of Early Childhood*, vol. 26, no. 1, pp. 33–8.

Raban, B., Ure, C. & Waniganayake, M. 2001, 'Multiple perspectives: Acknowledging the virtue of complexity in measuring quality', paper presented to the Warwick International Early Childhood Education Conference, London, March.

Rattler Information Series 1999, 'Advocacy', *Rattler*, 49, Spring, pp. 2–10.

Rattler Information Series 2001, 'Developing your centre's policy guidelines', *Rattler*, 58, Winter, pp. 15–18.

Rayner, M. 2001, *London's Children's Commissioner*, transcript of an interview with Julie McCrossin, Radio National, Australian Broadcasting Corporation, 22 Nov.

Razik, T.A. & Swanson, A.D. 2001, *Fundamental concepts of educational leadership*, 2nd edn, Merrill Prentice Hall, Columbus, OH.

Robertson, J. & Talley, K. 2002, 'Synchronistic leadership: Unleashing the power and passing on meaning, purpose and wisdom', *Child Care Information Exchange*, no. 146, Jul/Aug, pp. 7–10.

Robins, J. 1997, 'Separation anxiety: a study on commencement at preschool', *Australian Journal of Early Childhood*, vol. 22, no. 1, March, pp. 12–17.

Rockwell, R.E., Andre, L.C. & Hawley, M.K. 1996, *Parents and teachers as partners: Issues and challenges*, Harcourt Brace College Publishers, Orlando, FL.

Rodd, J. 1994, *Leadership in early childhood: The pathway to professionalism.* Allen & Unwin, Sydney.

Rodd, J. 1996, 'Towards a typology of leadership for the early childhood professional of the 21st century', *Early Child Development and Care*, vol. 120, pp. 119–26.

Rodd, J. 1997, 'Learning to develop as early childhood professionals', *Australian Journal of Early Childhood*, vol. 22, no. 1, pp. 1–5.

Rodd, J. 1998, *Leadership in early childhood: The pathway to professionalism*, 2nd edn, Allen & Unwin, Sydney.

Rosemary, C., Roskos, K., Owendorf, C. & Olsen, C. 1998, 'Surveying leadership in the USA early care and education: A knowledge base and typology of activities', in *Towards understanding leadership in early childhood context: Cross-cultural perspectives*, E. Hujala & A. Puriola (eds), Oulu University Press, Oulu, Finland, pp. 185–204.

Rosenbach, W.E. 1999, 'Mentoring: A gateway to leader development', *Training and Development Australia*, October, pp. 2–5.

Rosier, M. & Lloyd-Smith, J. 1996, *I love my job, but . . . : Child care workforce attrition study*, Community Services and Health & Industry Training Board, Melbourne.

Sarros, J.C. & Butchatsky, O. 1996, *Leadership: Australia's top CEOs: Finding out what makes them the best*, Harper Business, Adelaide.

Scarr, S., Eisenberg, M. & Deater-Deckard, K. 1994, 'Measurement of quality in child care centres', *Early Childhood Research Quarterly*, no. 9, pp. 131–51.

Schein, E.H. 1985, *Organizational culture and leadership: A dynamic view*, Jossey-Bass, San Francisco, CA.

Schoderbek, P.P., Schoderbek, C.J. & Kefalas, A.G. 1990, *Management Systems: Conceptual Considerations*, 4th edn, BPI/Irwin, Homewood, IL.

Schon, D. 1988, *Educating the reflective practitioner*, Jossey-Bass, San Francisco.

Schrag, L., Nelson, E. & Siminowsky, T. 1998, 'Helping employees cope with change', in B. Neugebauer & R. Neugebauer (eds), *The art of leadership: Managing early childhood organizations*, vol. 2, Child Care Information Exchange, Perth, pp. 232–5.

Schweinhart, L.J. & Weikart, D.P. 1997, 'The high/scope preschool curriculum comparison study through age 23', *Early Childhood Research Quarterly*, no. 12, pp. 117–43.

Sciarra, D.J. & Dorsey, A.G. 2002, *Leaders and supervisors in child care programs*, Delmar, Thomson Learning, Albany, NY.

Sciarra, D.J. & Dorsey, A.G. 2000, Developing and administering a child care centre. (4th edn) Delmar Publishers. Nelson Thomson Learning. Melbourne.

Sciarra, J. & Dorsey, A.G. 1979, *Developing and administering a child care centre*, Houghton Mifflin, Boston, MA.

Sergiovanni, T. 1984, 'Leadership and excellence in schooling', *Educational Leadership*, Feb., pp. 5–13.

Seyler, D., Monroe, P. & Garband, J. 1995, 'Balancing work and family: The role of employer supported childcare benefits', *Journal of Family Issues*, vol. 16, no. 2, pp. 170–93.

Sheridan, S. & Schuster, K. 2001, 'Evaluation of pedagogical quality in early childhood education: A cross-national perspective', *Journal of Research in Early Childhood Education*, vol. 16, no. 1, pp. 109–23.

Shimoni, R. & Baxter, J. 1996, *Working with families: Perspectives for early childhood professionals*, Addison-Wesley Early Childhood Education, Don Mills, Ontario.

Simons, J. 1986, *Administering early childhood services*, Southwood Press, Sydney.

Sims, M. & Hutchins, T. 2001, 'Transition to child care for children from culturally and linguistically diverse backgrounds', *Australian Journal of Early Childhood*, vol. 26, no. 3, pp. 7–11.

Sinclair, A. 1998, *Doing leadership differently*, Melbourne University Press, Melbourne.

Singapore Department of Statistics 1997, *Yearbook of Statistics*, Government, Singapore.

Singapore Ministry of Manpower 2002, *Manpower 21 Policy* [On-line, accessed 28 July 2002] (URL: http://www.mom.gov.sg/m21/index.htm).

Smith, A.B. & McMillan, B.W. 1992, 'Early childhood teachers: Roles and relationships', *Early Child Development & Care*, vol. 83, pp. 33–44.

Steers, R.M. & Black, J.S. 1994, *Organizational Behaviour*, 5th edn, Harper Collins College Publishers, New York.

Stehn, J. 1999, *The South Australian Curriculum, Standards and Accountability (SACSA) Framework: Intentions and Characteristics* [On-line, accessed 3 Aug. 2002] (URL: http://www2.nexus.edu.au/ems/sacsa/downloads/whats_new/intent_charac.html).

Stephen, C. & Wilkinson, J.E. 1995, 'Assessing the quality provision in community nurseries', *Early Child Development and Care*, no. 108, pp. 83–98.

Stone, S.J. 1995, 'Empowering teachers, empowering children', *Childhood Education*, vol. 71, no. 5, pp. 294–5.

Stonehouse, A. 1991, *Our code of ethics at work*, Australian Early Childhood Resource Booklets no. 2, May, AECA, Canberra.

Stonehouse, A. 1994, *Not just nice ladies: A book of readings on early childhood education and care*, Pademelon Press, Sydney.

Stonehouse, A. 1995, *Parents and caregivers in partnership for children*, Community Child Care Cooperative, Sydney.

Stonehouse, A. 1998a, 'If children are our nation's greatest resource, then why are we fighting to survive?' *Rattler*, vol. 47, Spring, p. 12.

Stonehouse, A. 1998b, 'It's sort of like being at home: Values and elements of quality in family day care', report for the National Family Day Care Council (Australia) and the Commonwealth Department of Health and Family Services, Canberra.

Stonehouse, A. & Woodrow, C. 1992, 'Professional issues: A perspective on their place in pre-service education for early childhood', *Early Child Development and Care*, vol. 78, pp. 207–23.

Storm, S. 1985, *The human side of child care administration: A how-to manual*, NAEYC, Washington, DC.

Sumsion, J. 2002, 'Revisiting the challenge of staff recruitment and retention in children's services', *Australian Journal of Early Childhood*, vol. 27, no. 1, pp. 8–13.

Takanishi, R. 1986, 'Early childhood education and research: The changing relationship', *Theory into Practice*, vol. 20, no. 2, pp. 86–92.

Talley, K. 1997, National accreditation: Why do some programs stall in self-study? *Young Children*, vol. 52, pp. 3, 31–7.

The Australian 2002, Employment Section, 2 February, pp. 21–3.

Thio, A. 1994, *Sociology: A brief introduction*, Harper Collins, New York.

Tinworth, S. 1994, 'Conceptualising a collaborative partnership between parents and staff in early childhood services', in *Issues in early childhood services: Australian perspectives*, E.J. Mellor & K.M. Coombe (eds), WCB, William C. Brown, Dubuque, Iowa; Melbourne, Ohio.

Toffler, A. 1990, 'November Toffler's next shock', *World Monitor*, vol. 3, no. 11, pp. 34–44.

UNICEF 1989, *Convention on the Rights of the Child*, UNICEF, Geneva.

UNICEF 1994, *The Progress of Nations*, UNICEF, Geneva.

UNICEF 2002, *The State of the World's Children 2002: Leadership*, United Nations Children's Fund, Geneva (URL: http://oecdpublications.gfi-nb.com/cgi-bin/oecdbookshop.storefront).

United Nations 1959, *The Declaration of the Rights of the Child*, United Nations, Geneva.

Vandegrift, J.A. & Greene, A.L. 1992, 'Rethinking parent involvement', *Educational Leadership*, vol. 50, no. 1, pp. 57–62.

Vesk, K. 1989, 'Child care at work: Privilege or prerequisite?', *Australian Institute of Management Journal*, no. 10, November, pp. 4–6.

Vining, L. 1994, 'Customer focused child care', *Every Child*, vol. 1, no. 2, pp. 16–17.

Wangman, J. 1995, *Towards integration and quality assurance in children's services*, Early Childhood Study Paper no. 6, Australian Institute of Family Studies, Melbourne.

Waniganayake, M. 1991, *Continuing professional growth: In-service training needs of child care staff in Victoria*, a report of a study commissioned by the Commonwealth Department of Health & Family Services, Canberra.

Waniganayake, M. 1998, 'Leadership in early childhood Australia: A national review', in *Towards understanding leadership in early childhood context: Cross-cultural perspectives*, E. Hujala & A. Puriola (eds), Oulu University Press, Oulu, Finland, pp. 95–108.

Waniganayake, M. 2000, 'Leadership in early childhood: New directions in research', keynote presentation to Professional Development Conference, Melbourne, January.

Waniganayake, M. 2001, 'From playing with guns to playing with rice: The challenges of working with refugee children', *Childhood Education*, vol. 77, no. 5, pp. 289–94.

Waniganayake, M. & Hujala, E. 2001, 'Leadership for the new century: What do early childhood leaders do? Critical reflections from Australia and Finland', paper presented to Association for Childhood Education International Annual Conference, Toronto, Canada, April.

Waniganayake, M., Nienhuys, T., Kapsalakis, A. & Morda, R. 1998, 'An international study of leadership in early childhood: The Australian perspective', in *Towards understanding leadership in early childhood context: Cross-cultural perspectives*, E. Hujala & A. Puroila (eds), Oulu University Press, Oulu, Finland, pp. 109–28.

Waniganayake, M., Morda, R. & Kapsalakis, A. 2000, 'Leadership in child care centres: Is it just another job?', *Australian Journal of Early Childhood*, vol. 25, no. 1, pp. 13–20.

Waters, J. 1998, *Helping young children understand their rights*, OMEP Australia, Melbourne.

Whitebrook, M. 1996, *California child care and development compensation study: Towards promising policy and practice*, final report, National Centre for the Early Childhood Workforce, Washington, DC.

Whitebrook, M., Howes, C. & Phillips, D. 1989, *The National Child Care Staffing Study: Who cares? Child care teachers and the quality of child care in America*, final report, Child Care Employee Project, Oakland, CA.

Wolcott, I. 1991, *Work and family: Employers' views*, Australian Institute of Family Studies, Monograph no. 11, Melbourne.

Woodhead, M. 1996, *In search of the rainbow: Pathways to quality in large scale programs for young disadvantaged children*, Early Childhood Development: Practice and Reflections, no. 10, Bernard van Leer Foundation, The Hague, Netherlands.

Wortham, S.C. 2001, 'Global guidelines for the education and care of young children: the work continues', *Childhood Education*, Fall, pp. 42–3.

Young, J.R. & Hite, S.J. 1994, 'The status of teacher preservice preparation for parent involvement: A national study', *Education*, vol. 15, no. 1, pp. 15–18.

Zbar, V. 1994, *Managing the Future: Unlocking 10 of the best management books*, Macmillan Education, Melbourne.

Zey, M.G. 1995, *The mentor connections: Strategic alliances in corporate life*, 3rd edn, Transaction Publishers, London.

Zigler, E.F., Kagan, S.L. & Hall, N.W. (eds) 1996, *Children, families and government: Preparing for the 21st century*, Cambridge University Press, New York.

Zollo, C. 1998, *Public Policy External Studies Guide*, University of South Australia, Adelaide.

Index